STORIES OF *EXTREME*
PiCKY EATING

Children with **SEVERE FOOD AVERSIONS** and
the Solutions that Helped Them

**Jennifer Friedman,
MS, RD**

PAGE STREET
PUBLISHING CO.

PAGE STREET
PUBLISHING CO.

First published in 2020 by
Page Street Publishing Co.
27 Congress Street, Suite 105
Salem, MA 01970
www.pagestreetpublishing.com

Distributed by Macmillan, sales in Canada by The Canadian Manda Group.

24   23   22   21   20   1   2   3   4   5

ISBN-13: 978-1-64567-192-3
ISBN-10: 1-64567-192-5

Library of Congress Control Number: 2019957341

Cover and book design by Molly Gillespie for Page Street Publishing Co.
Kids Icon © Shutterstock/NWM, Food Icons © Shutterstock/Volodymyr Leus

Printed and bound in the United States of America

Dedication

For my family, who taught me the value and joys of convening around the family table.

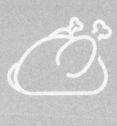

CONTENTS

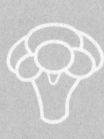
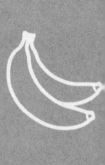

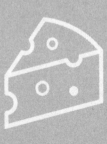
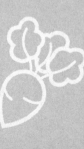

Introduction   7
Author's Note   11

PART 1: INDIVIDUAL CASE STUDIES   13

Chapter 1: Pouches, Please!—A Child Who Only Eats Fruit
and Vegetable Puree Pouches   15

Activity: Tastes Test   47

Chapter 2: Can't Touch That!—A Child Who Is Sensitive
to Everything   49

Activity: Sensory Play Bins   75

Chapter 3: He'd Like Fries with That—A Child Who Lives
on Nuggets and French Fries   77

Activity: Building Food Bridges   101

Chapter 4: Can I Get a Lunch Pass?—A Child Who
Can't Eat at School   105

Activity: Food for Fun   129

Chapter 5: Pizza Party—A Child Who Eats Pizza
for Dinner Every Night   133

Activity: Grocery Games   154

Chapter 6: Double Trouble—Picky Eater Siblings   157

Activity: Discovering Dips   180

Chapter 7: A Table for One—A Child Who Eats Alone   185

Activity: Comfortable Cooking with a Timid Eater   210

PART 2: INTERVENTION PLANS   215

Ten Tips for Successfully Introducing New Foods   216

Chapter 8: What Meals Should Look Like   219

Selecting and Serving New Foods   228

Chapter 9: Strategies for Introducing New Food
to the Most Extreme Picky Eaters   231

Chapter 10: Encouraging Kids to Eat and Interact with
New Foods   235

Endnotes   246
Acknowledgments   252
About the Author   253
Index   254

Introduction

How can we raise kids who grow up to become adults who eat well? This was one of the questions that drove my interest in nutrition ten years ago. The United States was facing what was dubbed the "obesity epidemic," and, as an unjaded, energetic twenty-something, I felt maybe we could turn the tide if we provided children with the right resources before they formed habits that would later be hard to break.

To this end, while earning my graduate degree, I spent time teaching nutrition and cooking lessons in New York City elementary classrooms. Interacting with food alongside children in the schools was a transformative experience for me. Very quickly I noticed that engaging with and talking about food came easily for the majority of the children I taught. Opportunity seemed to be the only obstacle standing between them and their willingness to sample a rainbow of fruits and vegetables or scoop up a dollop of homemade carrot hummus with a red pepper slice they cut themselves. But I also met another noticeable, yet smaller, group of kids who simply couldn't engage on that level. They were hesitant to touch, taste and even talk about the food we encountered.

That was the first time that I realized that eating is not something that we grow up intuitively knowing how to do. It was the first time I realized that there are some kids who experience genuine impediments to executing an activity that feels natural to so many of us and is so important to our well-being.

This reality reappeared in my work years later, when I began a private practice for autistic children. Kids on the spectrum are notorious for having poor diets, and I was aiming to help parents optimize diet to manage adverse symptoms and behavior. Yet when I actually sat down with families, I kept coming across one obstacle over and over: *My child won't eat that; he can't even sit at the table with us. She gags when I just talk about foods she doesn't eat. How do I possibly introduce healthy foods to my child who only eats a peanut butter sandwich cut into four perfect squares?* The realization I had while teaching nutrition had resurfaced, and this time it wasn't only interfering with school participation. It was a problem with profound ramifications.

So many of the children I met were facing genuine hurdles to eating not only a wholesome diet, but food in general. It became clear that I couldn't talk about improving nutrition without first resolving the issues that were impeding these children from having a comfortable relationship with food. Rather than abandon my mission, I morphed the goal from optimizing diet to breaking down the barriers that prevented kids from doing so. First, we'd address the eating problems, then we'd improve diet.

As I settled on this approach, the range of children I met began to grow. Extreme picky eating isn't unique to spectrum disorders, and it isn't a rare ailment. I now meet with a diverse population of children who have one thing in common: their inability to eat is interfering with their well-being and the well-being of their families. While the details of each child's eating difficulties are unique, the issues that extreme picky eaters face are universal. Therefore, the advice and strategies that I share apply to most kids who struggle with eating.

In the following pages, you will find a series of case studies interwoven with insight from my training, research and professional experiences. The principles of my approach to managing eating aversions are rooted primarily in Ellyn Satter's Division of Responsibility for Feeding; Cheri Fraker and Dr. Mark Fishbein's food chaining; and the value of hands-on sensory experiences, which is informed by several strategies, including Dr. Kay Toomey's Sequential Oral Sensory Approach to Feeding. I hope to shed light on how these practices can be applied and adapted to a variety of issues that manifest as a picky diet and give clarity to the hiccups and triumphs that arise as families adapt their feeding routines and work to transform their child's relationship with food.

The children that you'll meet in Part 1 represent a tiny fraction of the many "flavors" of eating struggles that children can face. I wanted to demonstrate the types of cases that I see most frequently and to reveal the serious impact that any eating anomaly can have on a child and their family. I also wanted to demonstrate that though on the surface it may not always seem like these struggles are debilitating, a child's inability to eat freely is always a tremendous stressor.

Even though we're meeting seven unique children with seven unique problems, you will see three themes repeated: environment, repeated exposure and hands-on exploration. While I do not advocate a one-size-fits-all approach, I do believe addressing these pillars provides children with the support they need to expand their diets. To that end, in Part 2 of this book, I share step-by-step strategies based on these themes that you can use to create your own approach to conquering picky eating at home. Additionally, at the conclusion of each case study chapter, you'll find instructions for a hands-on activity that was especially effective with that particular case. I use these regularly with clients in my personal practice, and I recommend them as vehicles for bringing some levity into what can be a challenging process.

I don't claim or seek to cure the type of eating difficulties that we see in this book, just as I don't envision any extreme picky eater ever eating all foods. Instead, I hope they can learn to eat foods from all food groups and do so comfortably. While I hope for children who struggle with eating to grow into adults who eat well, my priority is that they discover the pleasures of eating and sharing meals with others while enjoying the empowerment that comes with being able to feed their bodies what they need.

I hope you enjoy getting to know families that are similar to yours and share your frustrations, hopes, struggles and joys. Just as the approaches I use have helped them, I hope that the strategies and activities you encounter in these pages help revive your own picky eater's relationship with food.

A quick note: I use the word *picky* throughout this book to describe the type of eating behavior that we encounter. You will also see the terms *problem feeder*, *extreme picky eater*, *selective* and *particular*. We lack a term that adequately describes children who are not simply temperamental but who also do not have a clear diagnosable eating-related dysfunction. I don't feel that *picky* accurately describes the complexity of the struggles that the children featured in this book experience, but I settled on this word because it communicates something relatable about the diets and behaviors of the children you are about to meet.

Author's Note

The stories in this book are all true as told from my perspective. In order to maintain the privacy of the families I worked with, I have altered identifying details, including the names of the children and their family members. Despite these changes, the details of each case are depicted as accurately as possible from my recollection and perspective, and as documented in notes and video recordings.

Information in this book is solely intended to provide assistance to your personal efforts. It is not intended to diagnose or to be used as a substitute for personalized consultation, evaluation or treatment by a medical professional.

Part 1

INDIVIDUAL CASE STUDIES

CHAPTER 1

Pouches, Please!

A Child Who Only Eats Fruit and Vegetable Puree Pouches

Around the time that Jackson began to walk, he traded in his favorite sliced apples and teething biscuits for a diet of whole milk and colorful drinkable pouches filled with a blend of pureed fruits and vegetables. Nearly eight years later, nothing had changed.

When Jackson's mom, Julia, told me that her son ate nothing but cleverly packaged baby food, I thought she was exaggerating. Then she shared Jackson's food diary, a record of his intake over three days. She listed just one menu:

BREAKFAST: "Pear, Purple Carrot, and Blueberry" Plum Organics, 4 oz (113 g) + "Apple and Peach" Peter Rabbit Organics, 4 oz (113 g)

LUNCH: "Apple, Carrot, Squash" Peter Rabbit Organics, 4 oz (113 g) + "Apple, Sweet Potato, and Corn" Peter Rabbit Organics, 4 oz (113 g)

DINNER: "Pear, Spinach, and Pea" Plum Organics, 4 oz (113 g) x 2

SNACK: "Just Mangos" Plum Organics, 4 oz (113 g)

"He will also eat around two cups of one of the following with every meal and some snacks," she added, listing six easy-to-eat crunchy snacks, all some variation of Cheez-Its or Club Crackers. I learned that Jackson also drank 2 percent milk with every meal (his only source of protein) and on occasion would eat vanilla ice cream, vanilla milkshakes—vanilla only, not vanilla bean—and white cake icing.

That was it. Jackson had been eating little more than slurpable fruit and vegetable blends and milk for nearly his entire nine years of life.

Julia wasn't reaching out to me because she was concerned about Jackson's physical health. His growth was normal. His vitamin and mineral levels were normal. He didn't get sick any more than the average fourth grader. Instead, Julia wanted Jackson to get to the point where he could at least order one dish at a restaurant. She realized Jackson's limited diet would eventually impact his social life, and she didn't want to see him miss out or feel different from his peers. For the time being, Jackson was comfortable with where he was at with food, despite the fact that all of his friends and classmates ate a variety of foods. He didn't seem to mind sticking to his pouches while his friends shared pizza and fries at the water park that summer. Julia's worry was that one day he would.

Julia wasn't sure how they got to this point, and she was even less sure about how to move away from it. Jackson is bright and social and has a ton of energy. According to Julia, he "likes to be in motion" and would rather be moving than sitting. He excels in the bilingual immersion school he attends and gets along well with friends, babysitters and his grandparents who live nearby. Aside from his eating, the most exceptional part of Jackson's life is that he's an only child. Julia and his dad ended their relationship around the time that Jackson forewent his sliced apples, so it's been just the two of them for as long as Jackson could remember.

Jackson was a healthy baby. He had no major health issues and was developmentally normal. Julia says as an infant he was voraciously hungry, and she struggled to satiate his appetite with breast milk alone. He was fussy, but everything with his eating was fine. He didn't have reflux, constipation or any apparent food allergies or intolerances. Jackson moved on to solids without an issue, easily embracing new flavors and textures.

After a child's first flavor discoveries, which occur during the prenatal and early feeding periods, complementary feeding (the introduction of solids alongside breast milk or formula) is a significant feeding phase. It's at this time that young eaters acquire the skills and behaviors that ultimately inform their adult diet.[1] Eating is a learned skill. From birth through early childhood, children use their senses to make sense of the world around them. If you've ever witnessed a young child feeding themselves, you know that sensory exploration is a major component of how they learn to eat. Initial attempts at self-feeding are messy but important. Children derive pleasure as well as crucial information from exploring new tastes and textures with each of their senses. By touching, seeing, smelling, tasting and even listening, children develop trust and understanding of the new foods they encounter.[2] Direct contact with food helps children build positive pathways in the brain that let them know it is safe to engage with a food, thereby shaping the current and future choices they make about what they eat. These hands-on, messy eating experiences also promote self-feeding skills and are associated with reduced food neophobia.[3]

When Jackson started solids, he ate readily but resisted tactile engagement with his food. He never mashed his meal all over his face, hair, arms and hands as many kids do. Julia doesn't have a picture of him covered in cake on his first birthday. He would throw food, a clear sign he didn't want to eat or even be near it, but he never got messy. Even now, at nine years old, he liked things to be clean (to be fair, Julia did, too).

So, when Jackson transitioned to eating only his puree pouches, Julia wasn't alarmed or even surprised. The pouches were clean and quick, and it was easier not to fight with Jackson about what he ate. Plenty of babies enjoy those fruit and vegetable pouches, she reasoned. It was probably just a phase.

Jackson is headstrong. He participated in feeding therapy around the age of five, but he didn't make any long-term progress. His therapist suggested he and Julia transfer his purees to a bowl to provide more sensory interaction with his food and help him get used to eating meals that didn't come in a pouch. Julia and Jackson did as she recommended for a short time until Jackson decided it was too much work. Why did he need a bowl when his food came in its own container? Julia couldn't argue with his reasoning. Once he came to that conclusion, that was it.

Jackson is not the kind of child who is motivated to do something he doesn't want to do just to please others. He didn't see the need to add new foods or change his routine just because someone suggested it. "He's so stubborn," Julia said when she was telling me about feeding therapy. Still, she felt Jackson's eating was her fault in a way. She's spoiled him, she said. She never pushed him. She supported, and even promoted, his eating habits because they ultimately became convenient for her. Now Jackson is not only completely comfortable with how he eats but is actually scared to try new foods.

Stubborn is a word that many parents use to describe their picky eaters. While the trend is too common to be a coincidence, personality is not often the main cause of extreme picky eating habits. There's usually something more complicated going on.

Because Julia's divorce coincided with Jackson's change in eating habits, I wondered if the commotion, disruption and tension that often accompanies a relationship's end had upset Jackson, leading to a regression in eating habits and a stall in further development. But Julia told me Jackson was oblivious to her relationship with his father. They always sought to shield him from their confrontations. Plus, Jackson didn't display any signs of trauma from that time. He didn't even seem to remember it.

His early experiences with solids stood out to me. Avoiding the inevitably messy experience of eating is often one of the first indications of a sensitive sensory system. But it was Jackson's only sign. He had no issues with other triggers, like wearing scratchy fabrics, playing in sand or petting his three dogs. He still liked things to be clean. If a piece of food dropped on the floor during our therapy sessions, he was quick to pick it up and then immediately wipe his hands of any mess. Yet a compulsion for cleanliness didn't explain a lifetime of food avoidance.

In one of our later conversations, Julia revealed, almost as an afterthought, that Jackson suffered from strep throat and a series of sinus infections when he was younger. He was once on antibiotics eight times in four months and had his adenoids removed when he was five. She didn't remember exactly when the illnesses started. Was it around the time he was learning to eat? She couldn't confidently say. All she knew was that she was finally ready for her son to eat. As for Jackson, she assumed that he would get there eventually.

One of the unique things about Jackson's eating is that he manages to do it without really eating at all. Because most of his snacks essentially melt in his mouth, he barely has to chew. Because his pouches come ready-to-eat in an opaque container, he doesn't even have the opportunity to look at much of what he eats. These idiosyncrasies aren't unique to Jackson. They're common to those with severe food aversions and eating dysfunction. Kids who have strong visceral reactions to even the idea of eating might look for any way to avoid interacting with their food beyond what is minimally required. I've watched kids completely turn their heads with eyes averted when food is present or wiggle to sit backward in their chair to avoid visually connecting with a nonpreferred food on their plate. They're perfect fits for food that comes conveniently concealed in its own container.

Children who experience oral sensitivities or have oral motor deficits and therefore struggle to chew, swallow or manipulate foods in their mouth are known to have narrow diets that look a lot like Jackson's. These packaged foods that Jackson eats for snacks—a limited variety of chips and crackers—require minimal oral dexterity. Beyond that, they have the added bonus of consistency. Each package looks exactly the same. The food within that package is always the same. Unlike fruits, vegetables, meat and most food that is not manufactured in a facility, every single bite of the food within that package is exactly the same, too. The homogeneity and simplicity of these foods make them easy to eat and therefore appealing to those who struggle to do so.

Noticing these trends highlights the distinction between pickiness and potentially more concerning eating dysfunction. Picky eaters can be particular. They can have limited diets, and they can restrict their diets to the point of minimal variety. Yet, children with more serious barriers to eating are more likely to have true food aversions and rigid preferences due to a physiological impediment.

Despite the nature of Jackson's dietary preferences, chewing and visually tolerating food were not issues for him. He could orally manipulate any food texture he encountered in our sessions together and never showed signs of struggling to chew or swallow. Visually interacting with foods was also no problem. Yet maybe the consistent nature of his food choices and the minimal skill needed to consume them was telling in another way.

While Jackson's history of sinus infections seemed like an afterthought for Julia, it resonated with me. It's common for young children to reject foods they've eaten while sick. They have trouble distinguishing the eating event from the onset of their illness and come to associate the two. A child who vomits after eating spaghetti because they have the stomach flu might come to fear that spaghetti makes them sick. I wondered if, for Jackson, chronic discomfort, sore throats, runny noses and difficulty breathing had affected his eating from a young age. If eating was painful or exacerbated his congestion, it made sense he would gravitate to pureed foods, liquids and meltable solids like his favorite cheese puffs and buttery crackers, all of which require minimal effort to eat.

As to why he didn't outgrow his eating habits once his adenoids were removed, the simplest reason—really the only reason I could think of—is that he never had to. As bizarre as Jackson's eating was, his preferences were easy to accommodate. Julia never had to think about what to make for dinner or rush to cook his breakfast in the morning. It didn't even matter if Jackson was eating outside of the house. He could always bring his pouches to a friend's or on school trips.

Sometimes Julia did suggest Jackson try new foods. He was never interested. She offered him tastes from her plate or suggested something she thought he might like when they were out. He always declined. She never pushed him. Why would she? Jackson was growing appropriately. He did well in school. He had friends. He was happy. So Julia let him stay in his comfort zone.

Within that comfort zone, Jackson lacked a comparison point of more typical eating habits. Like many parents of selective eaters, Julia was used to preparing two separate meals. She kept Jackson company while he ate dinner on the couch with the TV on. TV helped him focus and he didn't use a plate or utensils, so sitting at the table never seemed necessary. Like many parents, Julia ate her dinner after Jackson went to bed. He was asleep before 7:30 p.m., and Julia appreciated the time alone to cook and relax. Like many parents, Julia wasn't a big breakfast person. Even though Jackson ate at home in the morning, she just had coffee. When it came down to it, she and Jackson rarely shared a meal. And because Jackson doesn't have siblings, he was generally eating breakfast and dinner alone.

As I continued to work with Jackson, his solo meals really struck me. Family mealtimes are incredibly impactful. Studies show that when teenagers share a family meal five times a week, they are less likely to try drugs or engage in underage alcohol consumption, enjoy healthier diets, report experiencing stronger family relationships and perform better academically.[4] Beyond that, meals shared between parents and children can directly impact a child's diet and food preferences. Research suggests that children are more likely to both overcome fear of new foods and try a novel food if they observe an adult eating it first.[5,6] Additionally, children model their parents' eating behavior and food intake and even adopt their parents' food preferences.[7] Ultimately, the repeated experience of eating together as a family, of continually seeing what and how others eat, can influence a child's diet quality, eating behavior and food preferences in meaningful ways.

Jackson missed a large part of the passive behavior modeling that children naturally experience when regularly eating with their families. Jackson, of course, didn't live in a food bubble; he was still exposed to food and witnessed others eating. He frequently saw his mom and grandparents eat, enough that he knew what their favorite foods were. He ate lunch in the school cafeteria, where he observed classmates enjoying everything from sandwiches to sushi and an array of fruits and sweet treats. The thing was, after years of eating pouches and drinking milk, Jackson also saw everyone else's eating habits as distinct from his. They ate *their* food. He had his. And that was okay with him.

Julia felt lucky that Jackson attended a small school where his teachers and peers were sensitive to his eating habits. She worried about what would happen in a year when his class flowed into a regional system and he encountered new kids who didn't know about his tendencies. That was part of why she reached out when she did.

I, on the other hand, worried about how comfortable Jackson would be shedding his idiosyncratic ways. Would he be willing to transform from someone who ate two things into someone who could eat anything? After nearly a decade of eating an unusually narrow diet, his eating habits had become more extreme than the more traditional picky eating that most children naturally outgrow. Anywhere from 6 to over 50 percent of children display selective eating behavior[8], and most parents report observing one or more problems with a child's eating at some point.[9] The large number isn't cause for alarm and it's not a growing trend. Picky eating is actually considered a normal part of child development. From the ages of around two to six, many children begin to limit the variety and quantity of the foods they eat. Babies who grew up devouring kale and roasted salmon turn into toddlers who prefer French fries and applesauce. Foods with bland colors and flavors replace more vibrant alternatives. The change in food preferences is thought to stem in part from a growing child's heightened taste buds, an evolutionary vestige that once helped increasingly independent children avoid bitter-tasting, potentially poisonous foods when they ventured away from their mothers.[10]

Alongside this, young children also undergo physiological and psychological developments that further complicate their willingness to eat. Growth stalls, contributing to decreased appetite and subsequent decreased caloric intake.[11] Psychologically, children enjoy a growing sense of autonomy, a preference for self-feeding and a new desire to participate in food selection.[12] Many children realize that mealtimes are one of the few areas of their lives where they can assert their free will. As newly independent agents, they'll reject foods they once willingly ate simply because they can.

In this early period of change and frequent food neophobia, distinguishing traditional picky eating from something more severe is challenging, in part because there is no formal definition of what either one looks like. Appetite and diet differ so drastically between individuals, and even within an individual's day to day, that it's difficult to measure when pickiness is occurring, when it's just a developmental hiccup or when it's something that warrants addressing.

Dr. Kay Toomey, a pediatric psychologist and feeding expert, created a framework to distinguish transient picky eating from what she defines as "problem feeding." Traditional picky eaters eat 30 or more foods. Their diets include foods from all food groups. They're comfortable having new foods on their plate—even if they don't eat them—and share a family meal. A problem feeder, on the other hand, eats fewer than 20 foods. These children do not enjoy foods from every food group and often reject foods based on texture or another distinguishing characteristic. Problem feeders often cannot tolerate new foods in their personal space and therefore commonly dine alone, eating a different set of foods than the rest of their family. Problem feeders also experience an increasingly limited diet, rejecting foods that they once loved and failing to reaccept them. Picky eaters, too, can reject former favorites, but they're more likely to welcome them back.[13]

Most picky eaters do outgrow their selectivity.[14] Appetites pick up. Their attitudes and taste buds change.

For many children, it is just a phase. But for some, it's the start of a lifelong struggle. Developmental delays, sensory sensitivities, medical conditions, food allergies and trauma can present real barriers to eating that preclude the natural return to more inclusive eating habits. When picky eaters grow up, yet fail to outgrow their selective eating habits for whatever reason, they can grow very comfortably into their identity as a picky eater. For Jackson, eating pouches was part of who he was. It was something people had come to expect. Letting that go could be hard. Who would he be if he wasn't the boy who eats pouches?

We had a lot of work to do with Jackson, but first I needed Julia. A positive, comfortable and distraction-free eating environment fosters healthy eating habits and forms the foundation of an ideal mealtime. Anxiety depresses appetite. Pressure backfires. Screens and toys interfere with interactions with food and distract a person from detecting their body's natural satiety cues. It's best for families to eat together at a dedicated eating location, where a child can sit comfortably and focus on their eating.

My first goal was to move Jackson from the couch. Julia and Jackson were to share one meal together a day. They'd eat at the table with the TV off, free of any other diversions that could detract from the eating experience and interfere with the social benefits of shared meals. Mealtime distractions like the TV often function as a coping mechanism. When children who struggle to eat are tuned into their favorite show, they give less attention to the discomfort they're experiencing. When eating feels comfortable, they're inclined to eat more. Jackson didn't need to eat more. He needed exposure to new foods and typical eating behaviors. He needed to see someone eat with a utensil, smell new food smells, hear the noises foods make when eaten and take in their different colors and shapes.

These exposures would prepare Jackson for his future encounters with new foods. At the same time, Julia's eating would provide an example, a model of what Jackson would be working toward. From there, when he was ready, he would have the opportunity to get comfortable with, and one day even try, new foods.

Adjusting how and where Jackson ate meals was Julia's job. Julia was so motivated and proactive in our time together that this foundational work happened seamlessly. Without hesitation, she adjusted her dinner schedule and even started eating breakfast just so Jackson had an additional opportunity to meet new foods every day.

Jackson also embraced their new eating routine surprisingly well. Julia told me Jackson "wasn't pleased" about turning off the TV at first, but that he actually liked eating meals with her at the table. He especially enjoyed making sure she put her phone away so they could enjoy the meal without distractions. Jackson's comfort with the new routine would serve him well. With shared meals as their new norm, mealtimes became an additional opportunity to incorporate the exercises Jackson would be learning with me.

A week after Jackson and Julia began sitting at the table for breakfast and dinner, we began our feeding therapy, a program I call Food Explorers, and I met Jackson for the first time. It was the middle of the summer. His skin was tanned and his blond hair bleached from the sun. He was quiet at first, and comfortable if not a little skeptical.

There's nothing wrong with a child who struggles to eat. Preferring certain foods doesn't make someone bad or different. Jackson needed to know that. He excelled in every other area of his life. His limited diet wasn't the one thing that made him flawed. It wasn't something that worried Jackson or made him feel ashamed. I didn't want the renewed attention on what he ate to change that. Before diving into our exercises, I emphasized that everyone struggles with something. In fact, most struggle with many things. I told Jackson that some kids need extra help with reading or understanding how to complete multiplication tables. Some need extra help with eating. Learning to eat new foods is like training your body to play a new sport, I told him. It might feel weird at first. It might be hard or a little uncomfortable. The more you practice, the stronger your muscles get, the more your body understands what it needs to do and the easier it becomes.

Wherever Jackson was at with his eating was totally okay for us. We were going to start at a place that was comfortable for him and move forward only as he felt ready. My job was to help him learn, but I would never push him beyond a place that felt comfortable. During our time together, I wanted him to be open to the possibility that eating could be fun, that exploring new flavors might be exciting. He might discover that he actually loves to eat a variety of delicious foods. At the very least, we'd work on helping him learn to be comfortable with new foods so he was no longer limited to his select few.

At some point soon, Jackson's body would need more nutrition than milk, fruit and vegetable blends and crunchy snacks alone could provide. Learning to eat new foods was therefore important for his physical health. But because food is an integral and ubiquitous cultural currency, the ability to tolerate even a limited diet was important for Jackson on a psychological and social level. Shared meals are not only an unavoidable part of human life, but they're also actually good for us. Research suggests that those who regularly share meals with others are happier and more satisfied with their lives than those who eat alone. Eating together facilitates social bonding and reinforces social networks, which makes it an important aspect of a person's personal and professional life and is known to enhance a sense of satisfaction with and connection to their community.[15]

Both logistically and socially, maintaining his unusual diet would become increasingly inconvenient for Jackson as he grew older and more independent. There would come a point when he felt embarrassed about what he ate, when his diet would hold him back or single him out. Would he miss out on vital bonding sessions with friends in his college cafeteria? What would happen when he was ready to date? Expanding his diet now would mean that he could share breakfast at a friend's house after a sleepover and avoid a crisis the next time one of his pouch flavors is discontinued. Down the line, a comfort with eating even just a few more conventional foods would mean that he could join colleagues at a restaurant and travel without a suitcase full of his favorite pouches. I wanted to focus on teaching Jackson how to eat so that he could more easily navigate these situations in the future. We'd focus on how to manage any food that didn't come in a pouch or package instead of working to add specific foods to his diet. Jackson felt okay with all of this, he said, and was ready to begin.

Before we did, I had to share my one rule. Jackson didn't have to eat anything he didn't feel ready to eat *yet*. A child who likes control and was skeptical of eating just about anything that didn't come in one of his six familiar pouches, Jackson visibly relaxed upon hearing this. I wanted him to know that I wasn't there to deprive him of his agency. He was still in charge of what he ate. He would progress as fast as his comfort zone allowed. Just as importantly, this announcement communicated a sense of possibility. Hearing his readiness to eat as something that could eventually exist opened the door to a future where he *would be* ready to embrace new foods.

As Food Explorers, Jackson, Julia and I were going to use our five senses to examine and discuss food. This method, based on the Sequential Oral Sensory (SOS)

Approach to Feeding developed by Dr. Kay Toomey, is a process of systemic desensitization that encourages children who struggle to eat to explore the different properties of foods in a progressive manner. By engaging a child's curiosity and inviting them to interact with food in a playful, nonstressful way, the program mimics the developmental process that children typically employ when learning how to eat.[16] It brings eating back to the basics for children who were unable to participate in that natural process for whatever reason.

The Food Explorers program would walk Jackson through progressive stages of interactions with food based on Dr. Toomey's six major Steps to Eating that inform the SOS Approach. Each of the six steps can be broken down into mini steps, which create a spectrum of food acceptance that runs from the least intimate form of engagement to the most. Tolerance, the most basic step required for successful eating, ranges from establishing a child's acceptance of food in the same room, to the acceptance of food at the table and is finally accomplished when a child can visually engage with food in their personal space, such as on their plate. To establish tolerance of a food in a child's immediate area, we start by describing the visual properties of food. What does it look like? What is the shape? Color?

When kids in Food Explorers have no issues with visual tolerance, they're quick to pick up the food to take a closer look. This puts them in the second phase of engagement, touch or tactile interaction. Familiarization with how food feels helps a child anticipate what this food might feel like in their mouth and between their teeth. This information makes the eating experience more predictable and therefore more approachable, so we explore whether a food feels heavy or light, bumpy or smooth, dry or wet. A child who is not yet comfortable enough to feel a food on their skin can use a tool, like a fork or even a preferred food, as a stepping-stone to help them explore tactile properties.

If a child is comfortable touching a food and is ready to move forward, the next level of engagement is exploring a food's smell. Smell is tricky for kids, and even adults, to describe. The first step is to identify whether a food has a small, medium or big smell before discussing specific olfactory properties. Again, some children will naturally notice a smell if they were comfortable enough to explore visual properties by holding a food up to their eyes. Others may not have issues tolerating smell in particular but are uncomfortable putting a food so close to their face.

Once smell is comfortable, we can move to tasting. Tasting, kids need to know, is completely different from eating. Tasting is no big deal if you just do a quick test with the tip of the tongue. We can practice how to flick our tongues quickly like snakes. As we did with smell, we can begin by rating the intensity of the flavor as small, medium or large. If the snake test didn't give us enough time to really detect the flavor, it's okay to experiment with tasting on different parts of the tongue, sucking the food or taking a longer lick.

The final sense to explore is sound: What sound does the food make when we crunch it between our teeth? Does it sound different if we take giant dinosaur bites on the back of our teeth or if we munch daintily on our front teeth like bunnies? Jackson and I would plan to conduct experiments to find out how the different types of biting and chewing could impact a food's sound, and even its taste, as Jackson was ready.

Conveniently, the task of listening to a food's sound on the teeth is the ultimate preparation for finally eating. Once biting is comfortable, we can explore the possibility of eating or at least getting closer to eating. If we're not ready to chew and swallow yet, we could start by chewing a few times and spitting the food onto our plates. Maybe we keep the food on our tongues and have a contest to see who can balance it the longest.

Moving through these phases to objectively identify

the sensory properties of food enables children to see food in a neutral light. A skeptical eater's neophobia can overshadow any potential for enjoyment. They're quick to notice everything that might be wrong about the food and cannot comprehend that something might not taste bad or make their bodies feel terrible.

Food Explorers have to shed their subjective impressions in order to discover the truth. We replace judgment words with objective ones and find more neutral descriptors for words with a negative connotation. Wet and shiny sound much less off-putting than slimy. Rough is more approachable than scratchy, soft more appealing than mushy. Even noting a food's very, very big smell is more pleasing than saying it stinks. By encouraging children who struggle to eat to replace their "I don't like it" reflex with objective data, the exploration experience creates the possibility for an enjoyable eating experience.

Discussing the findings from food exploration is powerful for highlighting a child's misconceptions about how a food looks, feels, tastes or smells. Often picky eaters have a myopic perspective and can obsess over minutia. They masterfully locate the one green speck on their pasta or can't see beyond the slight browning on a sliced apple. The discussion of a food's sensory properties becomes the opportunity to redirect these impressions. The observations are not untrue, but they do interfere with one's ability to embrace a diversity of food. Instead, conversations in Food Explorers include general reflections alongside the details. When we notice bigger picture findings, it's easier to generalize and create connections to preferred foods. Understanding that pears are crisp, crunchy, juicy and sweet like apples can help an apple lover feel more comfortable about eating something they haven't tried before. With more information, they are better able to anticipate what the eating experience will be like.

As I shared the steps with Jackson in our first meeting, I reminded him that along the way, he could always say, "No, I'm not ready." He could always stop. Julia and I might keep going, I told him. Observing our interactions could—and often did—show Jackson he could move further than he initially thought.

Jackson surprised us both on our first day as Food Explorers. We began the session with a familiar Club Cracker so he could learn the process without the stress of being around a new food. Jackson quickly got the hang of it and without hesitation moved on to a piece of cheese cut in the same rectangular shape as his cracker. He was pleased to discover that, like his cracker, the cheese was flat, yellowish and dry. Jackson described the cheese smell as "good," and when he took a snake taste by quickly touching the cheese with the tip of his tongue, he proudly proclaimed, "I like it." I did encourage him to find objective words to describe the taste as I hid my thrill with his comfort tasting and smelling the cheese, engaging more intimately with an unfamiliar food than he had in years.

Next up was hummus. The first thing Jackson noticed was that it had little black dots. Alarm bells went off for me. A more natural first impression would have been to notice the hummus's color, so I steered Jackson back to the bigger picture. The hummus was tan, not unlike the cracker and cheese. It was smooth, that he could see. He touched the hummus with some hesitation to confirm its texture before proclaiming that it had a very big smell. Julia and I agreed that the smell actually had a more medium intensity. Jackson wasn't convinced. We didn't argue. Instead, I explained that sometimes we experience new foods more intensely because our bodies aren't used to them yet. Part of Food Explorers was getting used to new foods and all of the sensations that come with them.

Hummus wasn't something that Jackson had ever

encountered directly because Julia didn't keep it in the house. It was a completely new food for him. I thought it might work because it shared a color with his snacks, which are pretty bland looking—mostly tan, white and the occasional orange—and the pureed texture was similar to his pouches. But Jackson actually struggled with hummus. I'd later see that wet textures and dips were some of his biggest challenges, a complete surprise given his affinity for the fruit and vegetable purees. Though Jackson didn't advance beyond smelling the hummus, he didn't lose his composure either. We complimented his reaction as well as his excitement to move forward.

We ended the first Food Explorers session with apple slices, dried apple chips and apple juice. Apple used to be a preferred food, so I thought a reintroduction might be comfortable and hoped that it could lead to acceptance. Jackson engaged with the apple up until it was time to bite. Even though he knew he didn't have to eat it, he said biting wasn't something he was ready to do yet. That was okay, I told him. Julia and I felt ready to move forward, though. When Jackson saw us make "bite art" by pushing our teeth through the apple slices just enough to leave an impression and create designs, he couldn't resist. Jackson bit into his apple a number of times and washed away the residue with sips of apple juice.

I left Julia with homework to add the foods we had explored to their breakfast and dinner rotation. When I checked in a few days later, Julia told me Jackson "LOVED" Food Explorers and was talking about it nonstop.

Jackson was motivated. He displayed a desire to progress and an interest in learning. When he told Julia he was interested in exploring mango, blueberries and Honey Nut Cheerios, we included these in a breakfast-themed Food Explorers session.

For a few weeks, we continued with basic Food Explorer sessions, which continued much like the first. Jackson's comfort grew. He liked knowing that he controlled the intensity of his interactions with food. He was eager to examine the day's food. He was still skeptical of many new foods, especially when it came to biting, but he enjoyed the learning process and was open to how he could move forward. When we noticed Jackson could use more time getting comfortable with new flavors, we made flavored water using fruits and vegetables we tried in Food Explorers. When he resisted progressing beyond a quick lick, we held contests for who could propel foods the farthest using our mouths. Jackson, like many kids, was more excited to participate in a potentially challenging activity when it was disguised as something fun, especially when that fun activity seemingly had nothing to do with eating. Flipping the switch from eating to playing rebranded the activity. It was no longer something that intimidated him. Instead, it was something he found to be both manageable and appealing. Of course, he did realize that spitting foods from his mouth would require him to actually put those foods in his mouth, the very action that he was resisting. But it was too fun for him to resist.

To supplement our work, Julia was conducting mini food exploration sessions on her own. She had also begun to serve Jackson some of what she was eating at meals. He was regularly interacting with scrambled eggs during breakfast and told Julia he wanted to continue working on them because they reminded him of movie popcorn, one of his preferred snacks.

Though Jackson wasn't yet eating new foods at meals, his comfort with them was growing. Julia told me that Jackson wasn't fighting with her about food (something he used to do when she asked if he would try something new) and that he was proudly sharing with his grandparents the progress he was making in Food Explorers. Sometimes, though, Julia felt like he was too smart and stubborn for his own good. One day he was eating apple slices, but then, she told me, "It was like he remembered he didn't have to," so he stopped and "just decided he wasn't going to try anything else." When he wasn't in the mood, he would tell her, "Miss Jenny said I don't have to try anything I'm not ready to."

We saw this in our sessions together, too. Jackson would confidently climb the Steps to Eating, picking a food up on his own before we even addressed its visual properties. He never had difficulty bringing a food to his face to assess its smell and was even quick to do a taste test. Chewing and actually eating, though, were different. He didn't struggle or display discomfort interacting with foods but would still adamantly resist the final stages. Julia and I didn't push him. Sometimes she would ask why Jackson couldn't move further. His response never changed: He just didn't want to.

In conjunction with our Food Explorer sessions, I was teaching Jackson nutrition basics: why the body needs food, which foods it needs and how each food group helps the body do something unique. We discussed that an ideal meal includes a protein, a fruit or vegetable and a starch. I hoped a rational explanation would serve as extra motivation for Jackson to expand his diet. Jackson understood the concepts well yet had a poor grasp of food groups. Julia told me that Jackson would come home from school some days telling her that a friend's lunch looked good. When she asked what the friend was eating, Jackson responded that he didn't know.

The day we had ranch dressing in a Food Explorer session really highlighted Jackson's deficits. He correctly assessed that the dressing was a little shiny and white with spots. As for touch, it felt slippery, wet and cold. He thought the taste and smell were huge, a reasonable assessment for someone used to nothing more flavorful than milk, Goldfish and fruit-sweetened vegetables. Jackson knew there was more to the ranch dressing's taste, but he couldn't find words to describe it further. When Julia and I suggested tangy, sweet and peppery, he agreed. Majority rules, after all. But it was clear that he didn't really know. Salty, sour, bitter and even sweet were words he recognized, but not tastes he could identify.

It was at this time that I realized how significantly Jackson's chronically limited diet had impacted him. After years of eating the same few foods and missing out on other food experiences, he ultimately lacked the vocabulary and knowledge to speak about food.

It was time to teach Jackson how to taste.

First, we needed a muffin pan. Next, labels: salty, spicy, sweet, sour, bitter and umami. Last, a sampling of food from each flavor family to fill each hole in the muffin tin. Sitting in front of a full muffin tin, a glass of water available just in case, we started tasting, ready to place an identifying label on the food when we recognized the correct flavor.

Distinguishing and recognizing flavors is a crucial skill for eating with confidence. Jackson lacked the ability not only to identify flavors but also to speak about his preferences in terms of taste. Understanding that something was too salty and therefore unpleasant tasting to him wasn't something he could do. This held him back from continuing to expand his diet. The Tastes Test sensory activity was one more tool that could help Jackson successfully navigate new foods.

With each flavor that we explored, we drew a connection to one of Jackson's preferred foods or another familiar food that shared the flavor. Chips were salty like his crackers. Honey and maple syrup were sweet like his pouches. Salt and vinegar chips were a little salty and a little sour, which was an unfamiliar taste.

Jackson realized that he liked salty and sweet foods the best. Spicy, sour and bitter tastes were very new to him, but that didn't mean he didn't like them. He just needed to keep trying.

The Tastes Test was intended to help Jackson learn to recognize flavors. It was also a lesson in empowerment. With more knowledge about food, Jackson would gain a new vocabulary to discuss and assert his preferences. He would feel empowered to make decisions about what to eat in the future. Over time, he could also learn how to adjust the way a food tastes to better meet his preferences by adding other flavors like sugar or salt.

Jackson used to cry when he saw a new food was on his plate. Now, according to Julia, he was very comfortable with new foods. "His language about food . . . is more positive. He's willing to touch anything. In the beginning, he really thought it was gross and he struggled. He wouldn't even have looked at a carrot, and he would have panicked if I had put a chicken nugget on his plate. Now it's not even upsetting him. It's been so good for him to explore new foods because he never did that as a baby," she told me at the end of one of our sessions.

We both embraced how far Jackson had come. Jackson could confidently move through the Food Explorer steps, licking, biting and even sometimes chewing and swallowing new foods in our sessions, but so far, he hadn't officially welcomed new foods into his diet. At meals with Julia, he tolerated new foods on his plate and didn't hesitate to interact with them, but he returned to his well-used "Miss Jenny says I don't have to eat anything I'm not ready to eat yet" instead of moving forward. Julia knew Jackson had the skills to eat new foods. She knew he could manage the experience and even enjoy it. She also knew how mulish her son was.

Controlling and *stubborn* are words I frequently hear parents use when describing a picky eater. Eating is one of the very few areas where children truly have agency and can assert their authority. Some really love to. I've seen children on the less extreme end of the picky eating spectrum who seem to have no underlying barrier to eating; they just love being in control.

Of course, Jackson's pace was nothing to be concerned about. He was progressing much faster than I had anticipated. Jackson had a lot of practice maintaining his routine. The well-learned habit was hard to break. And, even though Jackson was gaining new skills, he still lacked incentive to step outside his comfort zone on his own. Just as Julia knew before we started working together that Jackson was excelling in every area of his life and therefore resisted attempting to diversify what he ate, Jackson must have known that he was doing just fine without fully integrating into his diet all the new foods he was trying. If he was doing okay where he was, why change?

On one hand, Julia and I were confident Jackson had the skills to eat new foods whenever he was ready. On the other hand, we knew he could do it, and the longer he didn't, the more he was reinforcing his old ways.

It was important not to pressure Jackson. Pressure can work for some children in the moment, but it usually doesn't lead to sustained change in eating habits or a positive relationship with food. Julia and I both agreed, however, that Jackson would benefit from having his boundaries pushed just a little. At this point, Jackson's resistance seemed more psychological than physiological. Eating a variety of foods didn't seem to cause him physical harm or discomfort. He displayed no signs of issues with chewing, swallowing or even digesting food. He even reported liking many foods when he tried them for the first time. His sensory system was still fragile from lack of exposure for so long, but it was mostly his preconceptions that held him back. Despite months of practicing objectivity, Jackson's reflex response to so many foods was apprehension manifesting as "I don't like it."

With the goal of making eating seem more natural and comfortable to Jackson, we shifted the focus of our exercises to play using the mouth. We had tons of spitting contests, timed how long we could hold different foods in our mouths and experimented with the number of bites required to chew different textures. Instead of accepting Jackson's resistance, I offered coping strategies. If he had a negative reaction to eating something new, he could always spit it out or follow the bite with a sip of water or a preferred food. He could also pair the new food with a preferred one or adjust the flavor like we discussed in the Tastes Test. Finally, I highlighted over and over again that even when Jackson's body had a big reaction to a new food, even when he claimed he didn't like something, nothing bad ever happened. He was always okay. In fact, the experience was over quickly. He didn't have to fear trying new foods.

With these strategies in her back pocket, Julia amped up her dinnertime routine. She still didn't pressure Jackson to eat. There was absolutely no forcing. Instead, she suggested new ways that Jackson could interact with foods using his mouth and tongue. For example, he could chew a food twice and spit it out. He could hold it in his mouth for three seconds. Jackson still didn't have to, but most of the time he wanted to.

I didn't see Jackson for a few weeks due to vacations, a few colds and a busy back-to-school season. I caught up with Julia before our next scheduled session. "Jackson's doing really well!!!" she wrote to me in an email. "He even ate a cupcake at a birthday party!" There was no prompting, she elaborated. "He just ate the cupcake, like it was nothing. . . . His friends and I were all super excited!"

I was thrilled and I loved that Julia was, too. Jackson's eating the cupcake reinforced our suspicion that his stubborn tendencies were playing a role in his eating progress. He finally decided to eat something not because he had the skills or confidence, but because the decision was entirely his.

In our exercises, Jackson had gained information that would prepare him to eat absolutely anything, from cupcakes to carrots, when he was ready to do so. Eating is a skill, as I had explained to Jackson the first day we met, just like reading or completing multiplication tables. It wasn't surprising that Jackson chose to exercise his new skill with a fun and tasty treat among his friends. He was finally participating in a ritual his friends had been enjoying without him for years.

Julia's wish for Jackson to feel comfortable ordering something off of a restaurant menu was now a distinct possibility. Our work together was not done, though. We wanted to build on Jackson's success and continue building his foundation for broadening his diet.

As we progressed into the school year, I took a new approach in our Food Explorer sessions, focusing less on a logical sequence from his preferences and more on practicality when selecting foods to include in our exercises. I opted for foods that I thought he might encounter in social situations and could order from a kid's menu: chicken nuggets, pizza and grilled cheese.

Jackson continued to approach these foods tentatively. He wasn't ready to embrace the chicken nugget. He found the pizza much more appealing when he removed the cheese and wiped off the sauce with a napkin, and discovered that the crisp bottom smelled a lot like the crackers he loved. But he also continued to progress. The same day that he rejected the pizza's melted cheese he asked if he could explore a piece of sliced cheese. Julia and I gladly obliged, pleased he was initiating the opportunity for another exposure to cheese, a food we had included in sessions before. Instead of taking his time with the cheese as he had before, he picked it up and immediately took a bite. "It's good," he told us nonchalantly, taking another bite, as Julia and I smiled at each other, eyes wide.

Our sessions continued to be peppered with these pleasant surprises. Overall, Jackson was having an easier time engaging with the new foods we presented, but his most significant progress occurred when he took the initiative. He seemed to have his mind made up about what he would and wouldn't eat. As far as we could see, there was no rhyme or reason to his rejections and acceptances. It was a decision he made in the moment and he still resisted any encouragement or prompting.

Because of the progress we were seeing in our sessions, Julia was hopeful that the end was in sight. She believed at this point that Jackson's only barrier was his resistance. She wanted to allow him the time to abandon his resistance on his own, but she also suspected he would hold on to it as long as possible. They had a vacation planned in a few months, and she was wondering how Jackson would do if she "forgot" to pack his pouches. We decided it would be a reasonable experiment if Jackson continued to gain comfort with foods that he would be able to order in a restaurant. We selected grilled cheese as our focus, and Julia left with the plan to begin incorporating it into their meals.

After a series of postponed sessions due to cold-weather germs and busy holiday schedules, we finally reconvened several weeks later, directly after Jackson and Julia's trip. I knew from our intermittent check-ins that Jackson hadn't been making as much progress at home as Julia had anticipated. His biggest accomplishment had been requesting and finishing an entire cookie sandwich with a friend at the mall. Vacation turned out not to be the pouch-free experience Julia had been hoping for. Jackson's behavior was poor, and he rebelled the whole trip. He was unwilling to branch out from his pouches but did eat ice cream. Julia was frustrated because he was stalling and resisting when she knew that he was capable of more. This became even more apparent in our next session.

The timing wasn't ideal. Julia and Jackson had been having a difficult time together over a long school break that was coming to a close. Jackson had been pushing his limits, not just with eating, but in all areas. The session started off better than most. Jackson dove into a pile of cheese sandwich crackers, enthusiastically repeating, "I like cheese. I like these!" I was still on the grilled cheese theme and was optimistic about finally making some headway. Unfortunately, that was the most successful part of our session.

After dismissing many of the foods on his plate, ones we knew that Jackson was comfortable with, he began to tentatively poke at the cheese from his grilled cheese sandwich. Then we took it a step further and invited him to join us in eating the grilled cheese sandwich. He took a quick taste with the tip of his tongue, then tore off an impossibly small piece that he held on his tongue in his open mouth with no issue. Twice he munched it with his front teeth without a problem and willingly spit it out. But he refused to swallow. I saw how frustrated Julia was.

I tried to move on to the crust rather than push the issue. Jackson didn't mind touching the crust. In fact, he popped a sizable piece into his mouth, where he chewed it and then kept it for a long time, easily over two minutes. The bread was on his tongue. He was tasting it. It was likely melting in his mouth. All he had to do was swallow. He even admitted that he could, that nothing was stopping him. He just didn't want to. Ultimately, he spit out the chewed chunk of crust. Julia was indignant. Jackson's refusal felt calculated. It was clear the only barrier to his eating was the one he was creating.

The rest of the session was tense, but more consistent with Jackson's abilities. He ate several wisps of grated cheddar cheese, ultimately stating that he liked it more than Swiss, and he kept a whole piece of dried mango against his front teeth like a mouthguard for several minutes. He chewed a tiny piece, but, again, opted not to swallow.

That day Julia and I seemed to realize at the same time that continuing without any changes to our intervention would be futile. Jackson wasn't resisting the foods we offered because he couldn't eat them. He was resisting because he could resist, because he liked control. "For a while I didn't know if he was capable," Julia said to me during that session. "I thought that he had a real mental block. He doesn't. I know he doesn't. It's a control thing." I agreed. Throughout the session I was feeling that my work with Jackson was done. He *could* do everything that I was asking him to do, he just refused. We talked about potentially looping in a behavioral therapist. But first, we wanted to try one final approach that we hadn't yet explored.

Jackson was heading back to school in a few days for a short week. What if, I asked him, Mom started to pack some of the foods he had explored that day in his lunch box? For a long time, I had grappled with how to incentivize Jackson to eat new foods without depriving him of his usual meals and the reliable nutrients they provided. I hoped that with his permission and hopefully his input we could make some room in his lunch for new foods. They wouldn't be additions, but replacements. Running the idea by Jackson, asking him what felt okay and what he would like, I explained that we didn't want to do this to punish him or make him uncomfortable. Instead, we actually wanted things to be easier for him, to help him find more things that he enjoyed, to help him have an easier time with his friends and when he was older.

Despite his obstinance just minutes earlier, Jackson decided this was a plan he could get behind. He said he would help with the weekly menu and wanted to go grocery shopping with Julia. On the spot he agreed that he would welcome the cheese sandwich crackers, dried mango and grated cheese instead of his usual snacks. He said he'd eat them. We talked about eventually moving on to fresh mango, homemade cheese cracker sandwiches, nacho chips, sliced orange cheese and more when he was ready. Julia got excited, suggesting proteins and new fruits he could try.

As we reviewed this plan together, Julia proposed taking it one step further. For all of the previous significant weaning transitions in his life—potty training and giving up his bottle—Jackson was successful only when he went cold turkey. Julia didn't see him easing into anything at this point. "He's too defiant. He's just going to manipulate the situation," she said. Unless we didn't give him another option, she didn't think he was going to eat anything new. Jackson had just agreed to our new plan, and I didn't feel right about sending him to school without his pouches. Instead, Julia was considering eliminating pouches on the weekend in addition to providing Jackson with new foods in his packed lunch. She made a plan to grocery shop with Jackson. They'd pick out foods he felt comfortable eating, and they'd give the weekend experiment a go. This, she believed, was the push he needed.

When we touched base a month later, Julia was thrilled to share that since our last meeting, Jackson had consumed several grilled cheeses, a couple of cheese sandwiches, a chicken sandwich and one white bean.

Although Julia had come to me simply wanting Jackson to be able to order off of a restaurant menu, I sensed her goals had evolved. Once we had discovered that nothing but willfulness was standing in Jackson's way, Julia began to crave improvement in Jackson's daily intake. When he was eating nothing but pouches, the idea of him casually eating a grilled cheese was almost unfathomable. But once he began to comfortably explore foods he had avoided just months before, the potential for a new reality that included a more diverse and nutritious diet began to take shape. Now, the thought of Jackson eating out seemed like an auxiliary perk to his eating a more traditional diet every day. He wasn't yet there, but Julia could feel it. "He's perfectly capable," she told me. "It's whether he wants to or not."

We had seen that theme repeated many times over the months we spent working together, which is why I was shocked when Julia told me that Jackson was actually coming around. He told her one day that it would be nice if he could have one food that he could eat wherever he went. He wanted to focus on cheese sandwiches, he said, explaining that he liked them more than grilled cheese.

An individual's eating habits and preferences are perpetually evolving. Jackson's transformation, though many months in progress, was finally taking off in a big way. "A combination of things are coming together," Julia told me that day. "Jackson's getting older. He's getting to the point where he's going over to friends' houses more, and I think he's seeing it's kind of a pain to be the odd man out." Julia knew there was still room for improvement, but she also recognized that Jackson was heading down the path where his perceived limitations would no longer dictate what he ate. She knew that he could eat anything once he decided he wanted to, and Jackson was finally internalizing that, too.

Though Jackson wasn't yet ready to completely abandon the diet that he had grown accustomed to over nine years, he was finally comfortable making room for new foods. He wasn't necessarily growing out of his pickiness as much as he was growing into a new way of eating.

Every comfortable bite of a new food worked to erode his restrictive perceptions about the types of foods that he could and could not eat. His world was no longer comprised of his food and everyone else's. Everything was becoming available to him.

Julia told me that he spotted a bowl of crispy white beans at his grandmother's house one night. He was curious whether they tasted like crackers, so he ate one with the confidence of a child who had nonchalantly been trying new foods his whole life. Jackson might one day recognize the significance of his progress. For now, he was embracing it with the casual air of a comfortable, confident eater.

Activity: Tastes Test

This activity will help your child distinguish and learn about six basic flavors (sour, sweet, salty, spicy, bitter and umami/savory). Improved flavor recognition can help a hesitant child eat with confidence.

With younger participants, focus on building flavor familiarity. Once a child can recognize the different tastes, connect the tastes to commonly eaten foods. Identify individual flavors of new foods through a taste test. Then, organize individual foods by flavor or use the labels to mark each food's taste.

Older children can use the Tastes Test to draw associations with their current eating habits and hypothesize additional foods that they may prefer.

To take this a step further, experiment with flavor modifications by testing how the addition of sugar, salt, hot sauce or lemon juice to certain foods affects flavor.

What You Need
- Muffin tin
- 6 labels: Sour, Sweet, Salty, Spicy, Bitter, Umami
- 1–3 foods from each category:

Sour: lemon wedge, lime wedge, lemonade powder, vinegar, salt and vinegar chips, sour gummy candies, green apple, plain Greek yogurt, kefir, apple cider vinegar, sauerkraut, sour apple candies, red wine vinegar

Salty: table salt, potato chips, salted pretzels, soy sauce, seaweed chips, pickles, feta cheese, salted nuts, tortilla chips, olives, pepperoni, corn chips

Sweet: sugar, milk chocolate chips, honey, maple syrup, fruit jam, ripe fruit (such as banana, pear and mango), fruit-flavored candy, sweetened dried coconut, roasted sweet potatoes, caramel popcorn, dried fruit (such as dates, raisins and pineapple), caramelized onion

Spicy: hot sauce, radish, peppermint candy, mustard, arugula, salsa, strong-flavored breath mints, dried ginger, ginger sucking candy, spicy corn chips, spicy chorizo

Bitter: vanilla extract, unsweetened cocoa powder, raw Brussels sprouts, orange marmalade, citrus peel, walnuts, black coffee, over-steeped green or black tea, fresh cranberries, parsley, turmeric

Umami: miso paste, Parmesan or other aged cheese (grated or whole), jerky, anchovies, roasted mushrooms, roasted tomatoes

How To

1. Fill the openings of a muffin tin with at least one food from each of the flavor categories listed above.

2. Conduct a taste test. Use the labels to identify each flavor. Make it a game by seeing who can correctly identify the most foods. An alternative is to guess a food's flavor before tasting.

Take It Further: Group all items with the same taste. Discuss your child's preferences and identify foods that share their preferred flavors to try in the future.

CHAPTER 2

Can't Touch That!

A Child Who Is Sensitive to Everything

Our first call felt panicked. Claire had miscalculated the time change and was late for a meeting, but in the minute she had, she hastily revealed that her anxiety about her daughter's eating was quickly escalating. Ruby, weeks shy of her seventh birthday, had always been fussy with food, yet she had suddenly begun rejecting even her favorites and was losing weight. Ruby sometimes went through periods when she ate extremely little for days at a time and sometimes refused to eat at all. She was in one of these phases when Claire reached out to me. She felt time was of the essence. Not only was Ruby's already restricted diet shrinking, but her intake and her weight were too. Claire had to end the call, but she assured me the issue was urgent. When we finally connected later that day, Claire scheduled our first session for only a few days away.

In our first session together, I sought to learn more about Ruby's eating habits and history. Claire told me that as a baby, Ruby vomited frequently and had inexplicable reflux and gas. She eventually outgrew these symptoms, but never came to enjoy eating. In fact, eating actually seemed to be uncomfortable for Ruby. She liked only a few foods, mostly baked goods or packaged snacks, and ate those on repeat. On top of that, she had strong aversions to most foods outside of her usual rotation.

Because of Ruby's long-standing discomforts and difficulties, Claire had always worried about how and what Ruby ate. Whereas most parents contact me seeking support for their "picky eater," Claire initially told me that she was hoping Ruby could learn to "eat with more ease." She noted Ruby's tendency to gag when she encountered nonpreferred foods and told me that sometimes Ruby nibbled at her food with her front teeth instead of taking full bites. Additionally, it was concerning to Claire that Ruby approached all but her favorites with hesitation.

Although Ruby's declining weight was at the top of Claire's list of concerns when she first reached out, it quickly became clear that Claire's focus was more often on Ruby's limited and, in her opinion, unhealthy diet. Claire worried that Ruby didn't eat enough or enough of the right things. She was particularly fixated on what and how much Ruby was eating. She reasoned that if Ruby would just eat something new, she wouldn't have to worry anymore.

I agreed that Claire's concerns were valid. After all, the muffins, pasta, cookies and pancakes that Ruby was eating day after day lacked essential nutrients. Overall, Ruby had little variety and few foods with a robust nutritional profile in her diet. Despite Claire's concerns about the quality and quantity of Ruby's intake, the more I learned about Ruby's eating struggles, the clearer it became that her resistance to eating new foods wasn't the problem that needed fixing. That was just the surface manifestation of a deeper underlying issue.

Within just a few days, by the time of our first session, Ruby was back to eating more regularly and her weight had stabilized. With the urgency of improving Ruby's intake at least temporarily behind us, we could focus primarily on improving Ruby's relationship with food so that, as Claire had said so well, Ruby could eat with more ease and eventually come to enjoy a greater variety of nutritious foods.

When I shared with Claire my anticipated plan to help Ruby better understand and feel more comfortable around food, I sensed some resistance. She was ready to jump ahead. She agreed that Ruby had barriers to eating, but she felt strongly that the more pressing issue was to improve the quality of her diet. Claire thought that Ruby's learning to eat certain foods would solve Ruby's struggles and relieve Claire of her concerns. She believed we could address the source of Ruby's issues after we helped her eat a more nutritious diet. Claire was craving a short-term fix to what she saw as Ruby's biggest dietary deficits. However, not only would these measures not make a significant difference in the long run, but I also believed they simply wouldn't work. While intake and diet quality are important metrics when assessing a child's eating, they don't capture the complexity of factors that might coalesce into extreme picky eating. Simply suggesting a hesitant eater try new foods isn't effective. We had to first address the root causes of Ruby's struggles with eating before we could begin to see the improvements Claire was craving.

Ruby's distaste for the salads, steel-cut oatmeal and salmon that Claire wished she would eat wasn't random. Whatever was holding her back from eating these foods was what we would be addressing. From what I gleaned about Ruby's eating behaviors in just a few short phone calls with Claire, I suspected that Ruby had impaired sensory processing abilities that were impacting her eating. Food texture seemed to at least partially dictate her food selections. I noticed that she gravitated toward soft, easy-to-chew, mild foods. Ruby disliked the smell of most foods, and she found some seemingly benign tastes, like particular yogurts or crackers, unpleasantly potent. Also, Ruby had a hypersensitive gag reflex.

When Claire offhandedly mentioned that Ruby found many fabrics too rough, too scratchy or too restrictive and that she frequently fidgeted with tags in her clothing, I was even more convinced. These are hallmark complaints of a sensory overresponder. Overresponders tend to experience intense reactions to the world around them. It's as if they overprocess their environment. They can't adapt to the sensory input they experience and find it difficult to block it out. So, they wind up paying too much attention to things like strong smells or a scratchy T-shirt tag that other individuals can leave in the background.

I still wanted to observe Ruby's interactions with food and get to know her better before moving forward with this assumption, but from what Claire had shared, I suspected most of my work with Ruby would focus on improving her relationship with food from a sensory perspective. I planned to start with Food Explorer sessions. Regardless of Ruby's underlying eating issues, these sessions would help her learn to interact with new foods. At this early stage in our work, they would also help me observe how Ruby's senses responded to both new and preferred foods without the pressure or expectation to eat. If my hunch about her sensory defensiveness was correct, I anticipated that these sessions paired with hands-on desensitization activities could help Ruby's body feel more comfortable with the sensory component of eating.

Simultaneously, we'd also work on providing Ruby with strategies to manage her discomfort so eating could be more pleasant and find strategies to help improve her sensitivity to flavor. At the same time, I would be working with Claire to address the environmental aspects of eating so we could best support Ruby at home.

I first met Ruby for a Food Explorer session a few hours after lunch. Because we lived in different states, we conducted our Food Explorer sessions by video chat. Claire and Ruby were in Claire's office and I was in mine across the country. Seeing Ruby and Claire together was an interesting contrast. Claire was put-together, somewhat reserved and formal, dressed in monochromatic earth tones. Ruby, on the other hand, was a quirky little girl whose bubbly personality and curiosity radiated from her smile, her long strawberry blonde hair and her sparkly sweatshirt.

Before this meeting, Claire had stressed to me that Ruby was bright. She knew I worked with kids on the autism spectrum. Though Ruby had some learning difficulties—a teacher once suggested that she was "twice exceptional," a term used to describe those who are at once delayed and intellectually gifted—Ruby was smart and social. I didn't need Claire's warning to see that Ruby seemed wise beyond her years. Unlike any child I've ever worked with, she was curious about me and my life. She liked to chat with me during our video sessions, sharing details from her day and asking about mine.

Though Ruby was shy for a brief moment on our first video call, she quickly warmed to me, fascinated by our ability to meet despite our distance. I started the session by asking if Ruby had any idea why we were meeting. This was a chance to ease her in before introducing the food, but it was also important to me that we were all on the same page. She shook her head, so before beginning, I let Ruby know our plan. We were meeting to learn about food and how to make eating more comfortable. I had previously learned from Claire that Ruby liked ballet and horseback riding. I asked how she learned to do these complex activities. She told me that she practices both weekly. That's exactly what we would be doing with eating, I told her. Eating all foods is not something we're born knowing how to do. It's a learned skill that we need to practice.

Just as Ruby went to dance class, she'd be joining me for an activity called Food Explorers. At every Food Explorer session, Ruby, her mom and I would each have a selection of foods that we would examine like scientists. We'd spend time getting to know these foods and would simultaneously learn about why eating the different types of foods that we'd encounter is so important for our bodies. I told Ruby that some food helps our muscles, some our brains. Some give us long-lasting energy, while others give us a quick boost and then leave us feeling tired and low. We'd discuss which foods Ruby could eat to get just the right kind of energy that would help her do all of the things she loved to do. I continued to share that because our bodies get so much benefit from eating a variety of foods, we hoped Ruby could learn to expand her diet; however, eating during these sessions was optional. If Ruby wasn't ready to eat yet, no problem. We wouldn't pressure her. Eating new foods can be hard, I told her. It takes time to learn. I was confident that eventually she would enjoy a variety of foods, but in the meantime, she didn't have to eat something before she was ready.

I pointed out that Claire and I would be examining and learning by Ruby's side. We would all try anything that I suggested she try. Group participation would foster a sense of security as well as comradery. With the three of us sharing the same experiences, Ruby would see that she was not alone and that she was not being punished or singled out for her eating habits. Parental involvement is important when I work virtually because it bridges the inevitable disconnect that occurs when I'm not personally in the room with the child. However, I also ask parents to participate in our sessions because they are such powerful role models for their kids. Studies suggest that a parent simply offering a new food with a smile increases a child's willingness to eat.[17] Claire's joyful participation could therefore be the extra nudge to inspire Ruby to jump from touching and tasting foods in our sessions to actually eating them.

Ruby nodded along to my overview until it was time to get started. The first food we met was one that was familiar to her, a hollow apple cinnamon–flavored puffed snack that Ruby loved. Starting with a preferred food was intentional because many skeptical eaters shut down when they encounter a new food. Rather than introducing a novel food early on, we'd start with something doable to give Ruby an immediate win, and then we'd work our way up. Plus, the absence of neophobic barriers would allow her to learn the entire process of our exploration.

Ruby was so excited to encounter a favorite food that she barely paused for the preliminary interactions of smelling, touching and licking, and jumped immediately to the ultimate step of eating. After she devoured a handful of puffs and had regained focus, we met the next food of the day, apples sliced into stick shapes.

Ruby proceeded more cautiously. Apples weren't new. She used to eat them, but they were no longer preferred. Their familiarity was a main reason why I selected them. I also liked that Ruby would recognize the flavor from the cinnamon puffs and the occasional cup of apple juice Claire let her have. We had cut the apples into sticks to mimic the shape of Ruby's puffs. I hoped all of these details would create an easy entry point. But just in case, I asked Claire to bring ground cinnamon that we could sprinkle on the apples to add another point of familiarity.

Ruby picked up the apples with minor trepidation and correctly noticed that they were cut like "noodles" and looked similar to the puffs.

"How do they feel?" I asked.

"Ooh, slimy. Really slimy. Cold. Hard. Soft. Smooth," she said as she gingerly held a strip between the tips of two fingers.

Ruby's selection of the word *slimy* stood out to me.

Wet is probably what she was detecting, maybe some stickiness, too. Slimy is different than wet. It's ickier. Snails are slimy. Spoiled food is slimy. No one is excited to eat something slimy. I knew that Ruby would never be inspired to eat apples if their association to such an unappealing word cemented in her mind. So, I considered her response and asked Claire what she thought. "Not slimy," she said. No, the flesh was wet and cool. I agreed and pointed out that the skin felt different. It was smooth and dry. Ruby held the apple by the skin, a tactile experience that was less triggering for her, and explored the apple flesh again. She thought for a moment, brushing her finger along its surface. "It's wet," she finally agreed.

That first day and in future Food Explorer sessions, I sought to provide Ruby with alternative descriptions when I noticed her language take a negative tone. It's human nature to describe negative experiences with negative words, but when picky eaters speak disparagingly about their food, it only reinforces their aversion. That's exactly what I was trying to break down with Ruby. We didn't need to glorify food, but we did need to learn to see it neutrally. We were acting as scientists, after all, and scientists use objective language to describe their experiences.

To this end, I provided Ruby with a glossary of appropriate adjectives to talk about the foods we explored. The list provided words for each of the five senses she would use to assess the foods. I encouraged her to come up with her own initially. I didn't want to crush her creativity, and I was also curious to hear her first impressions, as they would provide insight into how she was perceiving the food and could help me continue to learn how to best address her barriers. But I did suggest she consult the list when she wasn't able to find the right words.

After we decided the apple was wet, not slimy, Ruby continued to tolerate the tactile interaction but was obviously not entirely comfortable with it. She made as little contact as possible and sat stiffly with her body leaning away from the apple stick. Still, she proceeded to smell, lick and—after sprinkling some cinnamon on top—even bite a small piece of the apple before spitting it out onto her plate, a coping mechanism I suggested if she wasn't ready to swallow. She rated both the apple's smell and taste as medium intensity, which seemed accurate.

Ruby did amazingly well with her first novel food in Food Explorers. I was proud of her for using all of her senses to explore the apple, and I was impressed with her willingness to participate despite her discomfort. She went on to engage only prudently with the other new foods in our first Food Explorer session, preferring to minimize her contact, careful that food touched only the tips of her fingers or tongue, and she was quick to wipe her hands as soon as she completed the necessary interaction.

Ruby's interpretation of sensory experiences, primarily her tactile interactions, continued to stand out to me. She found waffles to be "scratchy," but together we ultimately decided that they were a little rough and hard. She told me that strawberries and dried apples were both really bumpy. I agreed that they did have a lot of texture, but to me bumpy recalled the seam on a baseball. The strawberry had little bumps. The skin itself was soft and smooth, and then the parts near the seeds felt a little rough, like sand. The dried apple was soft and a little squishy. Its texture was uneven, but bumpy seemed like too big of a word to describe a dried apple.

As we went on, I was careful not to correct Ruby or suggest that her descriptions were wrong—after all, they were accurate in her mind. Instead, I wondered if we could find a better word. "Are you sure?" I asked her. "I can see how you might get that, but let's try again and see if we still really think that." Or I invited another opinion: "I wonder what your mom thinks." By providing her with the opportunity to rethink her answer and by using the power of numbers to suggest a more positive alternative,

I was hoping to rewire her perspective one adjective at a time. My intention was for Ruby to gain a new vocabulary while simultaneously developing more confidence with new foods. The two would help her eat more comfortably.

Ruby's tendency to pick intense words reinforced my suspicion that she was having intense reactions to the world around her. Sensory overresponders are often sensitive to touch and find particular sensations, like the feel of grass or sand, or labels and seams in clothing, distressing. They also appear to be more sensitive to tactile experiences in their mouth.[18] Oral sensitivities can contribute to increased fussiness with food. Research suggests this is one reason kids are prone to picky eating behavior. A comparison of children with and without a tactile defensive diagnosis revealed that those with sensitivities rejected more foods, ate fewer vegetables and refused novel foods more often.[19]

Similar findings have been confirmed in several other reports. In a 2009 study, a correlation between tactile sensitivity, food neophobia and decreased fruit and vegetable intake was observed in neurotypical children.[20] In another study, picky eaters ages five to ten years old were seen to have both taste and tactile sensitivities, which other research has confirmed is associated with increased food refusal.[21,22] These findings suggest that a higher sensitivity to touch translates to a dislike of eating particular foods and increased picky eating behaviors.

Ruby's language was telling, but it wasn't the only factor in our first Food Explorer session that reinforced my notion that her sensory processing was off. One look at Ruby's responses as she encountered both new and familiar foods confirmed that she had trouble managing the experiences on multiple sensory levels. She ate cautiously, taking measured and intentional bites. When she touched a food that rubbed her the wrong way, she splayed her hands as if she wanted to minimize contact and protect herself from something she perceived as threatening. Moreover, she was quick to wipe food from her hands or face, and she would wrinkle her nose, eyes wide, when considering an unfamiliar food.

Increasing evidence suggests that the sensory properties of food factor into the neophobic food response. It's a logical relationship: Eating is a rigorous sensory undertaking. The seemingly simple act of eating engages the entire sensory system, including the lesser known vestibular and proprioceptive senses, responsible for balance and movement, respectively. Eating is of course about taste, but taste is only one small part of a more complex experience. How food looks, smells, feels and even the sound it makes while we're eating can affect how we feel about that food. Difficulty processing sensory stimuli can therefore be a serious barrier to eating. It can impact one's willingness to eat and can result in a distaste for or an avoidance of certain foods, textures, colors and even entire food groups.

An estimated 5 to 16 percent of children have symptoms of impaired sensory processing abilities.[23,24] Those who experience impaired sensory processing have an atypical threshold for the amount of stimulation required to generate a reaction from the nervous system. Some children underrespond to their environment and require extra-strong stimuli, such as strong sensations or intensely flavored foods, to register a connection. Others, like Ruby, are hypersensitive to even subtle sensory input and find those same stimuli overwhelming.

Any hands-on exposure to new food would address Ruby's sensory deficits. Food Explorers targeted all of her senses explicitly; however, given the extent to which her sensory defensiveness seemed to be impacting her eating, I wanted to incorporate extra desensitization activities. I recommended that Claire incorporate sensory play activities into Ruby's routine.

Sensory play is an umbrella term for any activity that stimulates the senses: touch, smell, taste, movement, balance, sight and hearing. For instance, hands-on activities with crafts such as playing with playdough, finger painting, playing with toys in a sandbox or splashing around in a water table all count as sensory play because they stimulate various senses. Although a sensory activity may not involve eating directly, this work still prepares the body to eat. Regular participation in a sensory play program is associated with fussy eaters' increased willingness to consume more fruits and vegetables because engagement of the senses on this broad, holistic level develops neural pathways that support the architecture of the brain.[25] These developed pathways enhance one's senses, making it easier and more natural to use them all in a variety of healthy ways.

I've found that when children with eating difficulties and sensory impairments participate in regular sensory play alongside their work with me, they progress further and more quickly with their eating. Numerous studies support the benefit of sensory engagement to improve eating troubles. In one, children who were asked to feel different tactile stimuli and taste different foods exhibited an increased willingness to taste.[26] Thus, the opportunity for children to explore, play with and engage their senses is not only time well spent, but also a potentially crucial component to an improved relationship with food.

So, in addition to continuing our Food Explorer sessions, I assigned Claire and Ruby homework. At least twice a week I wanted Ruby to spend at least ten minutes engaging in some form of sensory play. I love using food as a medium, but it wasn't a requirement. I suggested Claire find a large container, like a storage bin, to create a sensory play space for Ruby. From there, the instructions were easy: fill the bin with a material that would stimulate a sensory response, like rice, birdseed, shaving cream or pudding, add in some toys or tools and let Ruby play and explore however she felt inspired.

Claire was hesitant about incorporating sensory play into their routine at home. She was still anxious about taking direct steps to improve the quality of Ruby's diet. She sat by as I incorporated options like apple-flavored toaster pastries that I know didn't meet her nutrition standards into Food Explorer sessions. She was willing to see how the sessions progressed. But playing with sand? She wasn't sure it was worth her time.

I acknowledged Claire's hesitation, but I didn't relent. Again, I reminded her of the complexity of Ruby's eating difficulties. I didn't think simply offering her kale in a new way would cure her pickiness. But I was confident that a multi-faceted approach that combined desensitization, hands-on interactions with food and, eventually, adjustments to Ruby's eating environment and schedule would.

We agreed on a month. For one month, Claire would trial sensory play. A month wasn't a long time to break down a lifetime of eating aversions, but after getting to know Ruby, I sensed that we would begin to see some progress in that time. If at one month, that was not the case, we could re-evaluate our plan.

At our next Food Explorer session a week and a half later, I was thrilled to notice that Ruby's perception and reception of food was evolving. This time when she encountered a slice of apple, she observed that it looked shiny and felt wet and a little sticky. Even though I could tell that she wasn't entirely comfortable engaging, she didn't ask for cinnamon before taking a taste with the tip of her tongue. The apple's flavor, she happily realized, was sweet. She nonchalantly took one small bite and then another—chewing and completely swallowing her first bites of apple in years—before moving on to the next items.

This session was breakfast themed. In addition to Ruby's favorite pancake strips and the now familiar apple slices, I included several new items: apple butter, the apple toaster pastry and turkey bacon, which was a formerly preferred food. Though Ruby licked the apple butter and toaster pastry, apples were the only food that she actually chewed and swallowed. The turkey bacon, a food she used to eat, was, she decided, "too black" to try. She was hyper-focused on the burnt pieces, and even though I showed her how to break them off, she wasn't ready to taste.

To my pleasure, during our third Food Explorer session, Ruby was more receptive to tasting. She took a little taste of a strawberry toaster pastry and thought it was okay. She noted it tasted sweet and tangy. I agreed, adding that the pastry part tasted bready. Then, Ruby moved on to strawberry yogurt. As she took a tiny taste with the tip of her tongue, I watched her face contort. Her whole body responded with a quick quiver. Ruby recovered and reported that the yogurt had a very strong flavor.

Claire had mentioned that ever since Ruby was very young, she complained that even mild foods tasted exceptionally bitter. From observing Ruby's list of preferred foods, I already knew that she preferred sweet flavors, and I tried to incorporate these into our sessions. I hadn't yet seen her react this way, and I wondered if I was off on my recommendation. To me, the yogurt was mild. It was sweet, fruity and just a little tangy. I asked Claire what she thought, and she agreed. When Ruby reluctantly took another small taste to test our hypothesis, she stood by her assessment. Again, she had to shake off the intensity of the taste. I got the sense that Ruby wasn't being dramatic. I also didn't think her barometer was off. By her reaction, it was clear that the yogurt was a very strong taste for her. That same session she nibbled a slice of red bell pepper. This, too, was very strong tasting, Ruby said. Again, Claire and I agreed it was sweet. But Ruby couldn't get on board.

At the end of the Food Explorer session, I brought

Ruby's reactions up to Claire in the few minutes that we touched base without Ruby. She told me again how Ruby was hypersensitive to bitter tastes. But that wasn't the only thing. She had noticed that Ruby also detected a bitter flavor in foods that others didn't. Because of the particular sensitivity to bitter flavors, I wondered whether Ruby might be a supertaster. It could be one explanation for the complete lack of fruits and vegetables in her diet (the closest she came to accepting a fruit or vegetable was drinking an occasional glass of mango nectar).

Supertasting is a genetic trait that causes the flavors of food, and in particular the bitter taste, to register more intensely than it does for most. The ability is attributed to the presence of extra taste buds and receptors on the tongue, and it is associated with a lower preference for vegetables and other bitter-tasting foods.[27,28] Even for children and adults who are not supertasters, we are naturally drawn to sweet foods and prefer to steer clear of bitter ones. Our bodies naturally crave sugar alongside salt, protein and fat, which are all sources of either essential nutrients or concentrated calories. The bitter taste, on the other hand, is one we're programmed to dislike. Since potential toxins, such as rancid fats, synthetic chemicals and poisonous plants, are typically bitter, the response is considered an evolutionary deterrent to our consumption of harmful substances.[29] Research suggests that young palates may be even more sensitive to bitter-tasting foods, a potential explanation for why kids stereotypically shun vegetables.[30,31]

There's no conclusive test to identify supertasters, but even a definitive answer wouldn't change my approach because there's no cure or management beyond adjusting dietary intake. Regardless of Ruby's tasting abilities, addressing her sensitivity to flavor was important. While a myriad of factors contributes to one's food preferences, taste has been identified as the ultimate determinant of what children eat.[32] We couldn't modify the number of Ruby's taste buds, but there were still simple solutions I could teach Ruby and Claire to make strong flavors more approachable.

First, we could try to modify flavor with thoughtful pairings. Sweet flavors counteract sour ones, making them more palatable, and vice versa. Salty and bitter flavors balance overly saccharine ones. Acid tempers salt. Roasting bitter vegetables transforms them into something decadently sweet, and bitter flavors mellow when paired with salty, sweet or sour flavors. These were techniques Claire and Ruby could learn.

Just as we added the cinnamon to Ruby's apple slices in our first Food Explorer session, we could adjust the flavor of other foods to make them more palatable for Ruby. When that yogurt tasted too strong on its own, I suggested Ruby pair it with a preferred pancake. Alternatively, she could add in a complementary sweet flavor like fresh fruit or jam. The red bell pepper would taste differently when cooked and when paired with Ruby's preferred hummus.

While Ruby might still not be entirely comfortable with the strong flavors even with these modifications, as long as she was willing to try, each taste exposure would help desensitize her palate. Sure, there still might be foods she disliked, but this would make it easier for her to tolerate unfamiliar foods and would prime her palate for new tastes. I advised Claire to try out some of these flavor pairings at home. At this point, she was incorporating foods that we used in Food Explorers into Ruby's meals and snacks. I recommended that she focus on foods like apples, which Ruby reported enjoying, but experimenting with how to modify flavors to make them more palatable was also a beneficial activity.

I enjoyed observing Ruby's evolution during our Food Explorer sessions and hearing about her progress from Claire. She had become open to tasting many new foods with the tip of her tongue, and her perceptions were becoming more neutral and accurate. I always incorporate foods that a child met in early Food Explorer sessions into new ones, sometimes in the same form and sometimes in a new form. Ruby's progress was particularly apparent with the foods that she had met multiple times. The first time we worked with peaches, she took one look, wrinkled her nose and described it as "a big orange thing." Her use of the word *big* stood out to me because I didn't serve Ruby a whole peach. She had a single slice. I could only assume that to Ruby, this brightly colored fruit was so unfamiliar and off-putting that it seemed giant.

To put the size of the peach into perspective, I asked Ruby to compare it to the other foods in that day's session: a carrot stick, a peanut butter cracker, a slice of cheese cut into a tall strip and a piece of pasta from a batch of macaroni and cheese. Looking at them all together, I asked her if it was really that big. Next to the other foods it became clear that while the peach was very orange, it wasn't that big after all. Ruby accepted this and moved on to exploring the rest of the items.

When the peach slice made a repeat appearance at our next session, Ruby was more open to engaging. This time, when she touched the peach with four of her fingers, she recognized that its flesh was wet and a little sticky. "Excellent," I responded as I reminded her that apples, which she had continued to grow fonder of, were also wet and a little sticky. "How is the peach different?" Ruby touched it again. It was softer than the apple. "Does it taste like an apple?" I asked. She successfully nibbled off a bite, chewed it with her back teeth and swallowed, declaring, "I can eat that." It turned out that the peach was sweeter than the apple.

I recommended that Claire incorporate peaches into Ruby's meals. In fact, because repeated exposure to unfamiliar foods is directly related to increased preference for those foods, Ruby would benefit from seeing any food that she encountered in Food Explorers on her plate.

Caregivers tend to be quick to accept a child's rejection of a new food, only offering something unfamiliar three to five times before concluding that the child simply doesn't like it. Yet research suggests that children generally need to meet a new food eight to fifteen times before finally eating it.[33] Real-world experience tells us that many kids will only just come to tolerate the visual presence or tactile experience of a new food after that amount of time and may take longer to warm up to something new.

I referenced this tendency and the importance of repeated exposures with both Ruby and Claire during our Food Explorer sessions. I needed Claire to see that Ruby required time to learn, that her progress would not be instantaneous. Similarly, it was important that Ruby was open to the possibility that her preferences would evolve. Though she had begun to make progress in her tolerance of novel foods, tastes, textures and smells, she would still encounter something new and instinctively proclaim, as so many kids do, "I don't like it" before even engaging with it. Instead of challenging her with the fact that she can't possibly know that yet, I shared the following anecdote with her and Claire.

I told Ruby that the brain is naturally skeptical of new things. When it sees something new, it assumes that our body won't like it. That's only because the brain isn't yet sure how to manage the new experience. If we always listened to the brain, we would never learn to like new things. This adjustment period can be hard, but it is just a phase. We can actually teach the brain to like new things. A group of scientists discovered that the more the brain encounters something new, the more comfortable it becomes. When they looked at how the brain welcomes new foods, they found that someone might need to meet a food eight or more times before their brain can decide whether they actually like it or not. Repeated exposures are therefore crucial for kids learning to expand their diets.

After hearing the story, did Ruby fully accept this and

go on to willingly and repeatedly taste new foods so she could train her brain to like them? No. But the important thing is that she did consider the idea that her opinions about new foods could evolve. She thoughtfully digested the story and reported that she was open to the idea of conducting experiments to learn more about how her brain worked. To support her in this journey, I gave her a tracker to record each time she tasted a new food.

The tracker provided Ruby with motivation to branch out. She was at an age where her incentive mattered. She was content with the current state of her eating. Her aversions and limitations didn't bother her, and she couldn't yet comprehend the long-term ramifications of her inability to eat comfortably. I had conversations with her about how her diet affected her body, how it provided her with the energy to dance, horseback ride and do everything else that she loved every day. Ruby was smart. She understood what I told her. But because she had yet to detect any limitations, the connection between what she put into her body and how she felt didn't fully resonate. The tracker, on the other hand, was something that she could wrap her head around.

Ruby's intake did not expand significantly after receiving the tracker, but in the following weeks she was proud to show me her progress at the start of our sessions. I got the feeling that knowing that she could record her accomplishments inspired her to take tastes that she would have otherwise passed on. As an example, remember the peach slice Ruby had first wrinkled her nose at? Within a few weeks' time, peaches had begun to make a regular appearance on the tracker, and Claire told me that Ruby was eating them with no hesitation or discomfort.

At the end of the Food Explorer sessions, I always spent a few minutes with Claire to review Ruby's progress and discuss other aspects of her eating. An important element I addressed early on was the environment in which Ruby was eating. At the end of our first session, I learned that Ruby was eating most of her meals alone. Meals took Ruby an hour to finish, and she was in the habit of eating every two hours. Initially, when I asked Claire about the details of where, when and with whom Ruby was eating, she tried to direct me back to the quality of Ruby's diet and the plethora of foods that she refused to eat. Again, Claire had a myopic view of Ruby's struggles, but I reinforced that we can't look at how or what a child eats in isolation because eating isn't one-dimensional. The environment—everything from where and when eating occurs, to the company, to the eating habits and mentality of a child's family—plays a significant role in a child's eating.

Despite Claire's resistance, I asked her if she could make some adjustments to Ruby's mealtimes and her eating schedule. I know that modifications to a family's mealtime routine can be a hard sell. Meals are more than a means to an end. They are products and reflections of one's culture and values. Beyond that, meals are such an ingrained part of a family's dynamic, and for most families, they happen the way they do for a reason.

Furthermore, adjusting the mealtime environment is not a quick fix for an extreme picky eater. Many experts believe that a supportive mealtime environment can be a sufficient intervention to stymie the progression of typical picky eating behaviors. A 2018 study found that children under the age of four who enjoyed family meals with a structured setting experienced reduced rates of food fussiness at the age of five.[34] Yet, for more extreme picky eating, the mealtime environment is often only one component of a larger approach.

I stressed to Claire that in addition to providing support, exposure and modeling opportunities, mealtimes could become a valuable daily opportunity for Ruby to implement skills she would acquire in Food Explorers into a real-life situation. I've heard too many stories about children who eat in a feeding therapist's office, but display no behavior change at home. My goal wasn't to teach Ruby how to eat more comfortably with me, but how to eat comfortably anywhere. To do this, we first needed to address Ruby's eating schedule because the mealtime environment was irrelevant if Ruby wasn't coming to meals hungry.

Most children need to eat every three to four hours, which generally translates to three meals and one to two snacks daily.[35] Ruby was eating eight times a day, at one-and-a-half- to two-hour intervals. That sounds like a lot of eating for a little girl, but Ruby wasn't exceeding her nutritional needs. Most of her meals were not substantial: almond milk and a cookie, a pudding cup or a handful of airy cinnamon puff snacks. So, even though she was incessantly eating, she wasn't eating well, and she was actually sabotaging her caloric potential.

In my experience, many parents of picky eaters, especially children with low appetite or weight, can be so eager for their child to consume more calories that they jump on any possible eating opportunity. What this often ends up looking like is a lot of snacking. Grazing can result in increased caloric consumption, but it is also associated with an excessive intake of calories deriving from added sugars and fats—unfortunately, not the kind of nutrition most parents are hoping for.[36] These nutrients are satisfying, but not filling. They don't provide the nutrition that sustains energy or satiates the appetite for long. Because of this, they actually perpetuate the snacking cycle. Kids will always seem hungry enough for an easy-to-eat snack but have a diminished desire to eat at mealtimes when more nutritious, but less appealing, foods are offered. Providing snacks is not intended to impede a child's intake, but ultimately, that tends to be what happens.

I didn't recommend that Claire abandon Ruby's snacks completely. Children do require frequent eating opportunities because of their small stomach size. Plus, with Ruby's recent episode of weight loss, I was hesitant to restrict her intake. The how and when of snacking is what needed modification. I recommended that Claire limit Ruby's intake to three meals and one to three well-timed snacks per day, which could not only help Ruby eat more at mealtimes, but might also make her more receptive to trying new foods. Claire was skeptical to make such a drastic change, so I shared with her the findings of a 2016 study that showed that eliminating grazing was the most effective intervention for improving weight gain in children.[37]

I also shared that the second most effective change was structuring meals and snacks. A regular eating schedule lets kids know what to anticipate and can condition their appetites to expect meals. Even though Ruby was eating what I felt was too often, she was eating at almost the exact same times every day. The consistency of her schedule was a plus. However, her tendency to eat alone was less than ideal. As a solo eater and the only child in her household, she was regularly served only her preferred foods, which meant she was missing crucial opportunities to expand her diet. The monotony of her meals reinforced her eating preferences and also limited any opportunity for her to learn to tolerate new foods.

Claire never considered Ruby's schedule or lack of mealtime companionship as potential factors in her eating tribulations, and she initially resisted my insistence on family meals. Cooking one meal for her family to eat together was one of her goals. But before now, she imagined eating together would come organically after Ruby's eating began to improve. This was true, but shared meals were also an important component of improving Ruby's eating. I told Claire that she wouldn't see the type of progress she was craving and certainly not at the rate she wanted if we couldn't focus on the environmental aspects of Ruby's eating.

When Claire ultimately agreed to try out family mealtimes, I shared my three basic parameters for successful and effective eating: 1) include at least one of the child's preferred foods, 2) provide at least one novel food on the table and 3) never beg, pressure or force the child to eat.

Including both new and preferred foods meant that Ruby would always have something to eat even as she was learning to tolerate new foods at the table. Avoiding pressure meant that Ruby could eat whatever and however she was comfortable. I stressed this with Claire because in an effort to boost Ruby's nutritional intake, Claire was in the habit of urging her to try new foods, particularly nutritious foods like Swiss chard, which Claire loved. The offerings came from a good place, but intention was irrelevant. Ruby wouldn't go near a green vegetable no matter how many times Claire offered, and I had a feeling Claire's imploring only reinforced Ruby's resistance.

Pressuring children to eat specific foods tends to have the opposite of the intended effect. A 2006 experiment assessing two groups of preschoolers demonstrated how counterproductive eating pressure can be. In the study, children were offered two soups every day, and though each group was encouraged to eat a particular soup, the children were ultimately allowed to make their own choice. After the study's conclusion, researchers found that the children had consistently selected the soup they were not implored to eat. The kids also made fewer negative comments about that option.[38] Ultimately, kids actually eat more, have healthier weights and enjoy a more positive relationship with food when they're allowed to eat without coercion.

Claire wanted what was best for her child. She knew Ruby would not eat new foods on her own, so in her mind, the only way to compel Ruby to try new foods was to ask her to do so. But that wasn't the case. Sharing meals together was a solution that would benefit them both.

Shared meals would provide Ruby with opportunities to meet the nutritious foods that Claire consumed while also observing how Claire ate them. Remember, I told Claire, she was Ruby's best role model. Best of all, shared meals provided a natural environment where Ruby could decide to try new foods when she was ready.

Because I knew that including Ruby in meals with Claire and Ruby's dad was a big ask, I didn't set any strict parameters on the frequency of shared mealtimes beyond suggesting a minimum of once per week. The more they ate together, the better.

One month into working together, we had established a comprehensive plan for Ruby. Together, we had completed three Food Explorer sessions. At home, Claire was beginning to space out Ruby's meal schedule and trying to eat as a family as often as possible. After seeing some progress, Claire had committed to continuing sensory play. Ruby had a vivid imagination and liked creating a kingdom in her bin filled with sand and dried beans. There wasn't any particular major improvement that inspired Claire to embrace sensory play; rather, it was a subtle shift that made it seem like everything was starting to come together. Ruby was tolerating new foods on her plate and was more inclined to interact with these foods, both in Food Explorers and at home with Claire. She was maintaining her weight and adjusting to her new mealtime schedule well, and her intake at meals improved. It seemed like Ruby had come to understand that new foods were going to continue to be a part of her life, and she was learning to eat and exist alongside them. So far, apples and peaches were the only new foods that she was consistently eating, but she was making more progress than she had in years.

After one more month together, Ruby had added a total of six new foods: turkey bacon, a new shape of pasta, hard-boiled egg whites and mini turkey meatballs dipped in tomato sauce, in addition to sliced apples and peaches. When I first met Ruby, she was eating less than twenty unique foods, not counting the many varieties of cookies or muffins that she embraced without discrimination.

Ruby's progress was still far from what Claire was hoping for. Ruby would stick to her preferred foods if given the option. At the dinner table, she still avoided vegetables and complex dishes with sauces or multiple ingredients, even though she knew she wasn't required to eat them. Still, I learned that she was eating more frequently with her parents. They served meals family style and though Ruby wasn't yet interested in eating, she was increasingly comfortable accepting small pieces of fish, chicken and potatoes on her plate.

I assured Claire that this trajectory was normal. It was understandable that Ruby first needed to tolerate the food before feeling comfortable putting it in her mouth. If Claire wanted to push Ruby along, I recommended that she incorporate Food Explorer exercises with new foods at the table. So far, they had yet to find time to complete the sessions independently at home, as I had suggested, and incorporating the practice into mealtimes would be an effective compromise. Claire welcomed this advice and added it to her arsenal of strategies to help Ruby.

I don't believe that there is a cure for picky eating, or that any individual with eating difficulties ever completely overcomes their barriers. I do believe, however, that there are strategies that can help kids and their families manage a picky eater's unease so they can learn to eat a healthy variety of foods more comfortably. The more Ruby and Claire could incorporate these strategies, the more Ruby's relationship with food would continue to evolve. Mealtime Food Explorer sessions were one such strategy, and the more we worked together, the more we found ways to move Ruby along.

Though I noticed improvements in Ruby's sensory

tolerance—she was more comfortable touching foods, spoke about the experience in less drastic terms and was less inclined to quickly wipe her hands—Ruby's hands-on engagement still required some prompting. When I knew that she could do something I told her so and went ahead with doing it myself, inviting her to follow along. She often did. When she seemed paralyzed by hesitation, I introduced a fun twist to encourage her to join me. These are strategies that can engage any child. When the interaction feels more like play and less like a challenge, fear often dissipates, making room for meaningful interactions. "Let's see who can make a bigger crunch," I suggested. "Could you make the food dance from side to side in your mouth?" Or, "Chew like a hippopotamus, just like me." When it was silly instead of serious, Ruby was more likely to participate.

Similarly, she responded positively at meals when Claire proposed: "Ruby, you can dip the meatball in your sauce. You can break the bacon into pieces before taking a bite." Ultimately, it wasn't just one thing that helped Ruby begin to expand her diet and feel comfortable around new foods. Her eating would be an ongoing evolution. But, with a combination of approaches, she had the support that she needed to continue to take steps outside of her comfort zone and learn to eat more diverse and healthful foods.

Activity: Sensory Play Bins

I suggest sensory play for any child who seems to have a sensory component to their picky eating. Activities that stimulate the senses with specific types of input can support sensory organization and reduce sensory defensiveness.

Food is always a great medium for play, but it's not always realistic and it's certainly not a requirement. Using everyday materials can be just as effective and might be more approachable for an extreme picky eater.

What You Need

- A large bin, such as a plastic storage container or plastic dish tub
- Filler materials (see below)
- Sensory play tools (see next page)

Filler Materials

Dry

- Dried grains like rice, oats, cornmeal or pasta
- Acorns
- Dried beans
- Cotton balls
- Pom-poms

Wet

- Soapy water
- Cooked grains like pasta, oats or cornmeal
- Pureed food like baby food, whipped cream, gelatin, yogurt or pudding
- Kinetic sand
- Frozen fruits and vegetables

Sensory Play Tools
- Plastic cups and bowls
- Measuring cups, spoons and scoops
- Silicone baking cups
- Plastic letters and numbers
- Cars and dump trucks

How To

1. Fill your bin with one or two filler materials. Borrow from the list above or try any of your own.

2. Provide toys or sensory play tools that will spark your child's interest and facilitate their engagement with the materials.

Ways to Play
- Scoop, fill and dump with cups, scoops, dump trucks and ladles.
- Write letters or draw pictures with fingers.
- Add toys such as trucks and cars.
- Hide toys in the bin.
- Put feet in.
- Use wet textures to make tattoos or face paint.

Take It Further: I recommend sensory play as often as possible. Playtimes can be as short as five minutes or as long as your child maintains interest. Encourage them to get hands-on, which allows them to explore the materials with multiple senses.

Sensory play is most successful when it's purposeful. Create a plan for the types of sensory bins you'll create and make a schedule with designated times for sensory play.

CHAPTER 3

He'd Like Fries with That

A Child Who Lives on Nuggets and French Fries

"Is this normal picky eating stuff, or is there something more going on here?" It was the question Ali had been debating for weeks before she reached out to me. Her two-year-old son Ryder had recently started to reject many of his favorite foods. He didn't have a robust diet to begin with and was now left with chicken nuggets, French fries and a small selection of starches like bread, crackers and baked goods. Ali had initially dismissed Ryder's limited diet and refusal to try new foods as typical. Picky eating, she knew, was a normal phase of development. But the more Ryder came to restrict his diet, the more his eating rubbed her the wrong way. To complicate things, Ryder was recently diagnosed with a spectrum disorder. Ali was in new territory and her stress levels were high. She wasn't sure if she should wait for the phase to pass or if Ryder's eating required intervention.

In our first discussion, Ali ran through a brief history of Ryder's eating from infancy to the present, hoping to give me a comprehensive picture of what we were dealing with and from where her concerns stemmed. As a baby, Ryder had reflux and was difficult to feed. His appetite and flexibility with food improved for a few months when he started solids, but overall, he had spent most of his life struggling to eat. She then provided an overview of his limited food list and asked what I thought.

Ali was really asking me if Ryder would organically outgrow his eating struggles. Even though nobody could accurately predict the trajectory of his eating behavior, that didn't change the fact that Ryder was having a difficult time now, and Ali didn't know how best to help him. Given Ali's stress and Ryder's recent restrictions, I felt that he would benefit from attention sooner rather than later. In my experience, the more time that picky eating tendencies have to become ingrained, the more difficult it is to change them and the more severe the eating behaviors become. Though Ryder's struggles weren't new, because he was so young at only two years old, his picky eating was still in its infancy. If Ali and I addressed his eating now before his fussiness had more time to take root, the process would be easier for them both.

Regarding whether Ryder's picky eating was "normal," it was hard to say without learning more and observing Ryder's eating face to face. Picky eating, traditional or otherwise, isn't a diagnosable condition with concrete symptoms. It exists on a spectrum of severity. From what Ali shared with me initially, I suspected Ryder's eating habits were not just a phase, but I didn't want to make a definitive assessment before learning more about Ryder's relationship with food and observing him myself.

Looking at a child's total number of accepted foods and their reaction when introduced to new foods is one of the initial ways I distinguish between typical and more extreme picky eating. Most typical picky kids eat a relatively wide variety of foods and tend to be flexible with those items as well. For example, even a child who eats a lot of chicken nuggets is likely to enjoy different varieties, not just one particular brand or shape. Additionally, many average picky eaters don't mind being around non-preferred foods as long as they're not pressured to eat them. On the other hand, those on the severe end of the picky eating spectrum can't handle encountering new foods—even seeing them, never mind having them on their plate—without a meltdown or strong reaction. Still, even with these distinctions, some children's habits may not all neatly align with one side or the other. Ultimately, I place less emphasis on a clear characterization than I do on understanding how a child's eating impacts their life, health and the well-being of their family.

I started with an assessment of Ryder's diet and observed his mealtimes in videos that Ali took of him eating to gain information on what was and wasn't working and where Ryder was struggling. This information would potentially give me insight into the causes of Ryder's struggles.

Ryder's diet was limited and homogenous. It contained fewer than twenty foods and lacked valuable sources of protein, dairy, fruit and vegetables. Though his chewing and swallowing skills were intact, Ryder almost exclusively ate easy-to-chew soft foods. Any variety of plain pancake, white bread, French toast or French fries was fine for him. He also enjoyed chocolate baked goods, especially cake, soft cookies and doughnuts. But he wasn't as easy-going with the rest of his preferences.

As for chicken nuggets, which he ate daily, he only accepted one specific shape from two different brands. Sometimes he ate applesauce, canned peaches or pureed fruit and vegetable pouches, the closest he came to accepting a fruit or vegetable. The only exceptions to his soft food tendency were saltines, Cheez-Its and Goldfish. Ultimately, Ryder was subsisting on a diet of highly palatable, mushy starches.

Ali also told me about the foods that Ryder used to eat, nutritious and diverse items like eggs, pasta and berries.

Since he dropped them, she felt that she had been striving and failing to get Ryder to try something new. However, when we sat down to look at what she was offering Ryder every day, we realized she wasn't actually serving him new foods. She just kept making meals she knew he would eat. It wasn't that she had never tried. Rather, after a few unsuccessful attempts, Ali concluded it was futile. She didn't like to waste time or food and the attempts didn't seem worth anyone's stress. As soon as Ali vocalized this, she saw the mistake. Devising a plan for how she could successfully introduce Ryder to new foods would be a major focus of our time together.

Too often I see parents of picky eaters set limits in their own minds about their child's dietary potential. A few rejections are demotivating. Multiple rejections are interpreted as fact. They think, *I guess they won't eat that!* and don't offer it again. It becomes a self-fulfilling prophecy. Remember, children might only come to embrace a new food after encountering it a minimum of eight times. In my experience, that number is actually much higher, yet most parents stop offering at half that many opportunities.[39]

Beyond that, many seem to forget that preferences and even rejections are not stagnant. Maybe Ryder truly didn't like the foods Ali offered at the time she offered them. Or maybe the bite size was too big. Maybe he was too full or too tired. Because kids are so fickle, it's always worth persevering. We never know when they might finally be receptive. Although we'd later address a comprehensive plan for introducing Ryder to new foods, I gave Ali a piece of preliminary advice: Ryder would never eat a new food if she didn't offer it.

As I watched the videos Ali had taken of Ryder eating dinner, two other peculiarities stood out to me. First, Ryder didn't feed himself. Instead, Ali fed him individual bites from a fork. When I brought this up to Ali, she told me that Ryder couldn't yet consistently manipulate a fork or spoon. It shouldn't have mattered. Most of Ryder's preferred foods were finger foods. Yet, for some reason, Ryder wasn't inclined to pick them up. Ryder also preferred individual bite-size pieces. For example, he resisted taking a small bite from a whole chicken nugget. Ali told me he had always been this way. His intake was better when someone fed him, so his parents always did. Because of this, it seemed like Ryder was a passive attendee at his mealtimes instead of the main participant.

Second, Ryder ate in front of a tablet. He was mesmerized by the screen, so engrossed in the videos he watched that at times it seemed like he forgot the reason for his sitting at the table. His intake was slow, and he rarely looked at the forkfuls of nuggets he mindlessly ate. With the combination of the videos and his parents feeding him distancing Ryder from his food, I was concerned that Ryder was missing important interactions that could help him expand his diet.

Neither of these issues was a telltale sign or cause of picky eating, but together the feeding issue and the tablet at the table very likely had a strong impact on Ryder's eating habits and preferences. Because they could interfere with his learning to accept new foods, these would be the first issues that I would address with Ali. Once Ryder's mealtimes were optimized so that he was more engaged with his food, I wanted to address diet quality. After learning that Ryder wasn't regularly encountering new foods, I knew that we also needed to establish a plan to bring more diversity into his diet. In short, first we'd work on Ryder learning to self-feed and on minimizing distractions at the table, and then we'd work on which foods Ali should be introducing and how she could best do so.

Both the tablet and Ali's feeding Ryder at meals became habits because Ali was concerned about Ryder's intake and she wanted him to eat better. Ali had little faith in Ryder's ability to eat what he needed to on his own. Part of this, she explained, was because Ryder's speech was delayed. Though he had no problem declining food, he never indicated that he was hungry. The other part was because Ryder just didn't really eat that much, especially when left on his own. Breakfast was his best meal. Many mornings he was ravenous, scarfing down several pancakes in just minutes, but sometimes he couldn't finish more than a few bites. Lunch, which he ate at daycare, and dinner were hit or miss. At most meals, Ryder required prompting to consume what Ali hoped was just a reasonable amount.

Ali was not alone in her stress or confusion about her son's intake. Most parents I work with ask about their child's caloric needs, usually concerned that they're undereating. The simplest way to determine whether a child is receiving the nutrition they need is by assessing their growth trends. If they're losing weight, not getting taller or falling off their growth curve, something could be off. But as long as a child continues their trajectory, there's no reason to worry about calories.

Ryder was a skinny kid, but he was growing appropriately and always had enough energy to make it through his day. Based on these facts and food logs that Ali had shared, I wasn't concerned about the adequacy of Ryder's intake. But Ali was. When I suggested we begin to work toward weaning screen time at the table and getting Ryder to eat independently, it became clear that Ali couldn't consider any changes to Ryder's routine until she was certain that he was eating enough.

In general, kids ages two to three require about 1,000 calories and up to 1,400 calories a day. I wanted Ali to have this information so she could start our work confident and calm, but I prefer not to focus on calories. I reinforced that this range is simply a generalization. Caloric needs vary greatly, depending on age, activity level and developmental stage. Gender might also play a role after three years of age. Because intake can fluctuate day to day and certainly child to child, I dissuade parents from calorie counting and putting too much focus on the numbers.

Instead, I advised Ali to look at Ryder's intake in teaspoons. In general, for each food group, children require a minimum of about one teaspoon for each year of their age at every meal. For example, because Ryder was two, he needed at least two teaspoons each of protein, starches and fruits or vegetables at every meal for a total of around six teaspoons of food per meal. If he didn't eat one of these food groups at a particular meal, he would likely need to compensate with a larger portion from the other food groups to feel full.

The teaspoon estimation can evolve as kids get older, as they're going through a growth spurt and especially if they become more active. For example, children ages four to eight can require a range of 1,200 to 2,000 calories a day depending on age, activity level and gender, which means their teaspoon portions will vary greatly. The helpful thing, I told Ali, is that kids are born with the ability to self-regulate their intake. Unlike adults, they haven't yet learned to overeat, eat when they're not hungry or even eat less than their bodies need. Because of the many factors that determine caloric needs, I suggest focusing on the larger growth trends and allowing kids to manage their own intake day to day.

Moving forward, I asked Ali to begin recording how much Ryder ate at each meal. This would help us see whether future adjustments to his mealtime disrupted his eating and, I hoped, would reassure Ali. When we first reviewed Ryder's intake a few days later, we discovered that Ryder actually was eating the right amount at dinner most nights. Breakfast and lunch were the anomalies, where he'd either eat significantly more or less. Overall, however, Ryder was consuming what he needed over the course of a day.

Despite the adequacy of Ryder's caloric intake, I still suggested that Ali start him on a powdered multivitamin. Although he was eating enough calories, the nutritional profile of Ryder's diet was suboptimal. Extreme picky eaters have increased incidence of dietary deficiencies, and picky eaters with spectrum disorders are at even higher risk.[40] Although it doesn't negate the necessity of consuming whole foods, a vitamin is a useful safeguard against these risks and would hold Ryder over as he learned to enjoy more nutritious foods.

Now that Ali was feeling better about Ryder's intake, we could move on to making modifications to his mealtimes. Ali fed Ryder and allowed him to eat in front of his tablet because she wanted him to eat better. Ryder did eat more efficiently and adequately with Ali's assistance, especially when he was distracted with a video. Yet the habits were not sustainable or productive. Ryder needed to learn to eat on his own without distractions or assistance.

I worried that, in addition to distancing Ryder from his food, Ali's feeding him toed the fine line between pressure and assistance. Although Ryder had no problems pushing the fork away or shaking his head no with his mouth firmly closed when he wasn't interested in eating, he was still sensitive to the fact that Ali was regularly prompting and encouraging him to take a bite. Ali's assistance might have been improving his intake in the short term, but picky eaters who are instructed, advised or coerced to eat become less inclined to and also experience decreased eating enjoyment.[41]

Similarly, despite the benefits of eating with a tablet, I believed that the distraction was impeding Ryder's growth as a more adventurous eater. Ryder hardly paid attention to his meal. Instead, he ate somewhat robotically, engaging with characters on the screen instead of the food on his plate. Again, my concern was that he was avoiding important interactions that could help him expand his diet. I've found that good intentions, such as improvements in caloric consumption, comfort or behavior, are often the driving factors behind the presence of a screen at the table. Research does indicate that distractions such as watching TV while eating are linked to higher energy intake, but not in a positive way. Eating while distracted is actually correlated with an increased risk of obesity and consumption of unhealthy foods.[42] More concerning for Ryder was the fact that mealtime distractions are also associated with a tendency to refuse and make negative comments about food.[43]

Ultimately, while the tablet and Ali feeding Ryder might have improved his intake in the moment, I believed he would be better able to regulate his own intake and would actually eat better overall without assistance and without a screen. When I asked Ali how she felt about letting Ryder self-feed, she admitted that she wasn't yet comfortable relinquishing her role. She worried that Ryder lacked the skill and stamina to eat what he needed on his own. Ryder's eating independently was an important point for me, but I trusted Ali's intuition and didn't want her to enter our work feeling uncomfortable. I needed her to buy in, but I also knew that Ryder would sense her stress, which could negatively impact his eating.

We ultimately settled on a compromise: As Ryder began to add more foods to his diet, she would yield her authority over his meals. In the meantime, I recommended that Ali start eating alongside Ryder, sharing his foods, even if just for a few minutes. Ali usually ate separately because she couldn't eat and help Ryder at the same time, so Ryder lacked an example of what eating on his own looked like. This way, Ryder would get a chance to model Ali's behavior without missing out on the nutrition he needed. If Ryder began to lose weight or demonstrate any other alarming behavior at any point, we'd reassess.

Concurrently, Ali agreed to trial screen-free mealtimes. Although Ryder had come to associate videos with eating, he didn't protest the first night when he sat down and his tablet simply wasn't there. "He doesn't mind," Ali reported, "but his attention is shorter." Without the tablet, Ryder engaged more with his food, even though Ali continued to feed him. In a video that Ali took of one of their distraction-free meals, I saw that Ryder was looking at his food and maintaining eye contact instead of looking over it as he did when he was watching the tablet. Ryder did tire at mealtimes more quickly. Because he was no longer zoning out for minutes on end, seeming to forget what he was doing at the table, his meals naturally became shorter, which was a side effect I had actually been hoping for. Before we started working together, he was eating for sixty minutes, which was too long. It's a challenge for most kids to remain focused on eating a meal for much longer than thirty minutes. Therefore, I typically encourage parents to aim for meals that last around twenty to thirty minutes, which is a reasonable amount of time for kids to concentrate and eat until they are full.

Now that we had alleviated Ali's concern about Ryder's intake and Ryder was beginning to eat without distraction, we could address his limited diet. Early in our discussions, Ali had revealed that she hesitated to even consider serving Ryder novel foods. After she realized that Ryder repeatedly refused to eat anything beyond his narrow range of preferred foods, she just stopped trying. She hated to waste food, and he didn't appear to be budging, so she didn't see the point. I had already discussed the need for multiple introductions with Ali, but she needed more direction.

Our plan for introducing new foods would have a few parts. First, we would identify strategic foods to incorporate into Ryder's diet that would fill current gaps in his nutritional needs (protein, fruits and vegetables). Then, I'd share direction on how to best introduce foods to increase Ryder's likelihood of accepting them. Finally, once we gained more information about how he responded, I would advise Ali on how we could further motivate Ryder to try the new foods. I expected this to take a few weeks and several sessions to get in place. First, Ali had to get the details. Then, I'd want to hear how Ryder responded before moving forward with a final plan.

Many parents approach me feeling lost and over-whelmed about what foods to introduce to their picky eater. "What is the best vegetable/meat/protein/fruit to introduce?" is a question I regularly receive, as if there's a universally picky eater–approved vegetable they don't know about. If only!

On one hand, there is no magic rule regarding the type of food to introduce. Any food is fair game. On the other hand, putting some thought and intention into which, and how, foods are introduced can yield better and speedier outcomes. Familiarity is a major factor in a child's decision to eat or not. Whereas new foods are more likely to generate a neophobic response, familiar and previously preferred foods have the benefit of established exposure and comfort. With that built-in comfort, the barrier to eating will be lower. That's why repeated exposures are so important to a child's acceptance of new foods. Thus, a simple way to decide which foods to begin serving to Ryder was to look to ones that he used to eat. Ryder used to love strawberries, pasta, mini meatballs, marinara sauce, macaroni and cheese, grilled cheese, apple slices, peas, yogurt and green beans. These formed our initial list of potential new foods to start offering to Ryder.

The next factor I wanted to consider was the family's eating habits. It's useless to encourage a fussy eater to acclimate to foods that the rest of the family doesn't eat just for the sake of diet expansion. So, I look to the family's preferences, routines and priorities. We might decide to target foods that will alleviate the food preparation burden and make it easier to serve one meal. Or we might focus on foods that make going out to eat easier for families who often do. For Ali, being able to make one meal that her family could share on the few nights a week they had the opportunity was a priority. Additionally, restaurant meals were a regular part of their life and therefore a regular source of stress for her. Knowing that Ryder could order something other than French fries would eliminate much of her concern.

Ultimately, we decided to focus on tomato sauce, peas, green beans, strawberries, grilled cheese and macaroni and cheese—though any foods from the list, and really any foods at all, were still fair game. We selected the fruits and vegetables in part for their nutritional value and because they could easily be incorporated into meals the family would eat. The grilled cheese and macaroni and cheese could be ordered from many restaurant menus and would increase Ryder's protein intake.

Although Ali felt better having a curated list of novel foods, she had offered Ryder new foods before without success. We had previously discussed the need to provide him with more than eight tastes of new foods, so she knew repeated introductions were vital to Ryder's eventual acceptance. I also shared with her general guidelines for ensuring those exposures were effective.

First, because children are more likely to try new foods when they're paired with familiar foods and flavors, I recommend serving a novel food alongside a preferred food.[44,45,46] Next, I suggest offering a small portion of only one new food at a time. Keeping portions small and avoiding serving two novel foods concurrently can decrease overwhelm and eliminate the sense of pressure to eat that kids might experience. Children have decreased willingness to eat when faced with too many novel food choices.[47] Kids are conditioned to think that they have to consume all of what's on their plate, so sitting down to a large portion of a new food can feel like an unmanageable task. A small bite, however, can seem doable. Keeping portion sizes small has the added benefit of minimizing the inevitable waste that comes with feeding a child.

For a child with severe food neophobia, I might suggest starting off with a portion of a new food that is as small as a grain of rice. It's an extremely small serving, but that's exactly why it is so effective. Less sensitive children, on the other hand, should be able to manage meeting a larger portion, about the size of a pea or grape, of a new food. The goal is to start at a manageable size and increase the portion size as the child's comfort grows. I recommend first increasing the bite size (so increasing from the size of a grain of rice to a pumpkin seed and so on) and then total portion size (five seed-sized pieces, for example) until the child is eating an age-appropriate serving.

I felt Ali could start somewhere in the middle for Ryder. If he was trying macaroni and cheese, she could place a teaspoon-sized portion on his plate. When Ryder was self-feeding, he could take what he wanted from this portion. Yet, when Ali was serving Ryder, I suggested she offer him only one noodle at a time. If either of these portions seemed overwhelming—if Ryder couldn't tolerate seeing them on the plate, for example—I recommended Ali scale back.

I shared this with Ali in a session with just the two of us and sent her off to try it out for two weeks, until our next meeting, when I planned to share additional strategies to encourage Ryder to try new foods. Ali reached out to me in the time between those sessions to share the first win. Ryder welcomed strawberries back into this diet without so much as a blink of an eye. The first time Ali served him one at breakfast, he picked it up and popped it into his mouth as casually as if he had been doing so all along. This was a double win. Ryder both fed himself and ate a food he hadn't had in months.

Introductions to peas and pasta were less successful. Ryder initially accepted a piece of pasta from Ali and held it in his mouth for a moment before seemingly realizing that it was unfamiliar and spitting it out. He didn't even make it that far with peas. He didn't want to try them. I wasn't discouraged. Ryder's initial rejections didn't mean that he didn't like the foods, only that he wasn't ready to eat them *yet*.

We're accustomed to thinking that eating is binary—eating or not eating. But it's not that simple. Learning to eat can actually happen in stages. Not swallowing a food is not a setback or an indication of failure. Amid Ali's discouragement, I reminded her of Dr. Kay Toomey's Steps to Eating, an outline of more than thirty progressive interactions that children may need to engage in before ultimately consuming a novel food. Toomey identifies six basic steps—tolerates, interacts with, smells, touches, tastes and eats—and breaks each into micro-stages that children take as stepping-stones leading them from one phase to the next. For example, tasting could include licking with the tip of the tongue, or, more intimately, biting, chewing and then spitting out.[48] If Ali could recognize that even Ryder's seemingly unproductive interactions, such as looking at or mouthing a bite of food, were progress, then she would feel better about her efforts and be better able to track and celebrate Ryder's progress. I reminded Ali to continue offering all three foods and urged her to be open to Ryder's process of learning to eat.

Over the two weeks before our next meeting, Ali was relieved to learn that Ryder tolerated the new foods on his plate. Although he wasn't yet eating anything other than strawberries, he interacted with his novel foods when prompted. Observing videos of their meals, I noticed that often, when Ali was feeding him, Ryder would distractedly accept a bite of a new food and hold it in his mouth for a few moments before spitting it out when he realized it wasn't a familiar nugget or fry.

Two weeks ago, Ali would have found this disheartening. Now she knew these interactions were productive steps in the right direction. She understood how significant it was that Ryder was comfortable having food in his mouth, even for only a few seconds, and that this was his way of working to eventually become comfortable chewing and then finally swallowing.

The daily exposures to formerly preferred foods got Ryder off to a promising start, but I had a suspicion that his compliance was largely a side effect of his detachment when eating. Ryder was still in the habit of avoiding his food. His eating was not an interactive experience, but a means to an end. From the videos that Ali took of Ryder's meals, I noticed that he still tended to make little contact with his food, rarely looking at it or touching it beyond what was minimally required to eat. Ryder was getting more exposure when Ali encouraged him to feed himself, but she was still feeding him the majority of his meal. For the next phase in our plan, I wanted to create an opportunity for him to engage more with his food so he could learn to feel comfortable eating it.

When they're first learning to eat, babies make friends with new foods by playing with and exploring them with all of their senses. They sniff, smear, squeeze or smush an unfamiliar food not as an avoidance tactic, but as a way to prepare their bodies to take their first bite. Ryder didn't do these things. Because Ryder preferred solids and because Ali had always fed him, he didn't get messy with food. Even now when he was increasingly managing finger foods like chicken nuggets on his own, food rarely veered from his mouth. Ryder ended meals just as clean as he was before them.

Ryder's missing out on these formative interactions was not the cause of his eating struggles. It was more likely a symptom of whatever was driving them. Due to Ryder's food preferences and his tendency to avoid interacting with his food, I suspected that Ryder had some level of sensory defensiveness. In my experience, selective eating almost always has a sensory component. Children with tactile defensiveness or other sensory dysfunction are known to refuse more foods, have fussier behavior and eat fewer vegetables than children without sensory issues.[49] And although sensory processing problems are not universal in the autism population, 78 to 90 percent of children with a spectrum disorder have impaired sensory processing abilities.[50,51]

I believed that exercising Ryder's senses and creating opportunities for him to engage in hands-on experiences with food that he had missed could help him overcome his aversions. Therefore, to help Ali and Ryder begin to incorporate hands-on experiences, we scheduled a session to engage in food play. Regardless of the extent of Ryder's sensory impairments, encouraging hands-on experiences through food play could only improve his relationship with food and enhance his likelihood of one day eating a greater variety.

Food play is meant to be a fun and organic experience. Of course, the ultimate goal of food play is to promote eating new foods, but children are most open to the experience and do best when food play is conducted outside of mealtimes so there is no confusion about the motive. When eating is off the table, stress levels are low, food is more approachable and the door opens for neophobic children to experience novel introductions in more appealing ways. Effective food play stimulates all of the senses and naturally progresses through the Steps to Eating. The key is to keep food play fun. Anything that encourages a child to smile while touching, smelling and getting to know a food is an effective use of food play.

Ryder's first session had a mix of familiar and novel foods. His familiar foods included dinosaur chicken nuggets, penne pasta and marinara sauce. The novel foods were carrot and potato French fries, an orange cheese stick and baby carrots. We set up our first session in Ryder's play area and scheduled our meeting between his usual mealtimes so he wouldn't be too hungry or so full that he wouldn't be interested in tasting.

Ali and I sat alongside him and began to play. We dipped the French fry into the sauce and used it as a paintbrush to create a winding red path on the silicone place mats we had set up in front of each of our chairs. I picked up a nugget and trotted it along the path. Ali followed with her nugget. We invited Ryder to participate. "Does your dinosaur want to dance on the red road?" we asked him. After considering for a minute, Ryder picked up his dinosaur to join us. We continued to play in the road. Ali and I made dots with our fingers and then added a few pieces of penne to create bridges.

I decided that my penne was too dirty, so I cleaned it off with my tongue. Ryder watched for a moment and turned away. He was not interested. It seemed that tasting was too big of an ask, so I tried to make the next interaction less intense. This time, I brought the penne up to my lips like a horn and started to blow into it, making some music. Ali did the same, looking to Ryder as an invitation. We could tell that he was interested, but he was hesitant to touch his still saucy pasta. I showed him how he could clean it with his tongue. He was still not interested. Instead of pushing, we offered him the option of a napkin to clean it off or a plain piece. He went with the latter and began to blow through his penne horn as well. This was a big accomplishment for Ryder. He had unknowingly consumed a taste of macaroni and cheese when Ali fed it to him, but pasta was not something he had touched with his own hands in months.

Ryder timidly continued the session. We used the carrots as drumsticks to add to our musical ensemble and ripped off pieces of string cheese to make necklaces, bracelets and mustaches. Though Ryder didn't nibble anything unfamiliar that day, he did engage with his food in ways that he never had before and employed all of his senses in the process.

Ali was pleased with Ryder's participation, but disappointed that he hadn't eaten anything new. I reminded her that Ryder hadn't avoided eating. Instead, he was just working up to it. Eating was likely to come after multiple exposures to and positive encounters with new foods. Through repeated positive interactions, Ryder would build the confidence and comfort to finally eat when he was ready.

Ali and I continued to lead food play sessions together for the next several weeks. Although the play was fun, it took Ryder some time to get into it. He wasn't only encountering new foods but also engaging in more hands-on contact with food than he had ever experienced before. Our sessions together never were Ryder's most productive tasting experiences. He tasted more at mealtimes but explored food more during play, which underscored the importance of his doing both.

Soon, Ali felt comfortable leading the food play sessions independently. I recommended continuing them at least weekly, but ideally more often. When I checked in to see how food play was going a week or two after we stopped our shared sessions, Ali admitted that she was struggling to fit it in. I didn't want her to stop focusing on distinct food play sessions; however, food play at mealtimes is also valuable. For one thing, it mimics the typical exploration that infants engage in at mealtimes. Second, play schemes at meals can encourage interactions that might not otherwise happen when a child avoids a novel food, as Ryder often did. The regular exposure to nonpreferred foods during mealtimes was still not Ryder's favorite. Because he was not inclined to explore or taste even most formerly preferred foods on his own, Ali could add on play interactions to push Ryder along further than he was independently motivated to go.

With ongoing food play sessions and repeated exposure to novel foods at mealtimes, Ryder became increasingly comfortable engaging with food in dynamic ways. Several weeks after introducing food play, he was feeding himself more often, both with his fingers and with utensils, and he was showing more interest in the contents of his plate, signs that Ryder was moving up Toomey's Steps to Eating. Weeks earlier, these sorts of interactions were not in his realm of possibility. Now, they were becoming his norm.

In addition to offering food play at home, Ali continued to introduce formerly preferred foods at mealtimes using the three strategies we had discussed. Ryder was making good progress. He continued to accept strawberries and was also tasting peas and macaroni and cheese more frequently. However, Ryder wasn't budging on other foods like yogurt, meatballs and apple slices, despite multiple encounters both at mealtimes and in play sessions. So, I set up a session with Ali to share one final strategy: food bridges, also known as food chains.

Because Ryder's preferences were so ingrained, I thought we could use them to our advantage. I envisioned using commonalities in Ryder's preferred foods as a platform to introduce new ones that share similar features. Children eat the foods they eat for a reason. It could be the flavor, texture, temperature, look or a combination of these qualities. When these preferences are carried over to novel foods, children will be more inclined to taste and like what they're tasting.

We already knew that Ryder preferred easy-to-chew, somewhat mushy foods with a uniform texture that didn't change with chewing. When Ali and I sat down to look for patterns in Ryder's diet, we realized, too, that he liked warm foods and that his favorites were generally beige or brown. As for size, Ryder had an easier time managing food in small pieces as opposed to larger ones he had to bite from. Although Ryder didn't have any strict shape preferences, Ali was certain he would be partial to anything that resembled a French fry. Finally, Ryder appeared to prefer mild flavors.

With a clear picture of the qualities that attracted Ryder to his favorite foods, Ali and I created a list of potential new foods for Ryder that I was really excited about: starchy, soft vegetables like steamed and roasted sweet potatoes, carrots and turnips; vegetable and sweet potato fries; fish sticks and breaded white fish; hummus; vegetable nuggets; and baked apples.

The key to successfully building off of a child's preferred foods is not simply to offer similar completely novel foods. Instead, I suggest changing the preferred food in a small but meaningful way by making alterations to the taste, texture, look or temperature. Each change serves as a small piece of a bridge that guides a child away from their preferred food and closer to novel ones. Ultimately, the progressive changes pave the road to an expanded diet. A study measuring the success of food chaining found that after three months, it helped extreme picky eaters increase their food repertoires by an average of twenty foods.[52]

The same principles that Ali used to introduce formerly preferred foods applied to the ones she would be presenting as bridges. We selected fish nuggets, a new brand of chicken nuggets and sweet potato fries to try first because of their similarities to Ryder's favorite foods. The fish nuggets looked almost exactly like the chicken nuggets he ate daily, and like his nuggets, they had a crispy exterior and a mild, light-colored interior. The sweet potato fries had a familiar shape and texture. Only their color and taste were unique. Importantly, the nuggets and sweet potato fries were ideal springboards with a lot of potential for further bridging. Once Ryder incorporated fish nuggets into his diet, I had visions of moving on to fish sticks and eventually whole, breaded fish. He could make similar transitions with the chicken nuggets, eventually coming to enjoy breaded chicken cutlets, chicken tenders and one day chicken Parmesan and roast chicken. After he welcomed sweet potato fries, he could advance to butternut squash and carrots.

Ali introduced the bridge foods during mealtimes using the same principles that she had been using for formerly preferred foods: offering just one new food at a time, pairing a new and a familiar food and starting with small portions. She also had food play as a backup technique if Ryder ignored the new foods.

It turned out that Ali was overprepared. Without hesitation, Ryder accepted a piece of a frozen sweet potato fry that was very similar to his preferred brand of French fries. He even picked up and ate a few pieces on his own. Ali's inclination about the fry shape seemed to be right. He accepted the new chicken nuggets just as openly. But the fish nuggets were less of an easy sell. Ali served them to Ryder on a fork cut into bite-size pieces. The first several times she served them, he accepted one or two bites that he mouthed for a moment before spitting them out. Ali told me in a weekly check-in that she was discouraged. Although she had only tried a few times, the exposures felt futile. Still, she continued to offer fish nuggets regularly alongside Ryder's usual chicken nuggets. She encouraged him to play with them at meals and Ryder usually participated. In a few videos, I saw that Ryder followed Ali's lead. He gave the fish nuggets kisses, tapped them on his nose and swam them around in front of his face. But when Ali popped a piece into her mouth, telling Ryder that the fish nugget got lost in the cave, Ryder stopped. His fish had a better sense of direction and preferred to steer clear of caves.

After three weeks' worth of introductions, Ali began to wonder whether Ryder just didn't have a taste for fish.

I reminded Ali that everyone's—and especially kids'—taste is prone to evolving and can be acquired through repeated exposure. Not entirely convinced, and certainly frustrated with wasting so many fish nuggets, Ali nevertheless agreed to continue serving them. She sent me a short email a week after our conversation. Ryder's teachers reported that he had eaten fish sticks at daycare.

This wasn't the first time we had surprising news from Ryder's teachers. Over the past three months or so of our working together, Ali was receiving periodic reports that Ryder was no longer consistently ignoring his school-supplied lunch and was actually trying new foods at daycare. Over a period of just two weeks, he reportedly tried apple, pear, celery, red bell pepper, cherry tomatoes and a tuna sandwich. A little while later she learned that he ate part of a cheese sandwich and part of an orange. The fish sticks were just the latest in his list of accomplishments.

After learning about the fish sticks and having seen the improvements that Ryder was making at home, Ali began to believe that Ryder was turning a corner. Progress was slower than she had anticipated, but it was certainly there. Ryder was considering, touching and consuming more variety than he had in months.

After several more weeks of continuing our strategies and introducing even more new foods, Ali was noticing meaningful improvements. "He's more willing to try things, especially fruit and especially at daycare. He's eating new foods now and before we started with you, he wouldn't even touch something new. Now he's really comfortable with new brands, and he's definitely eating different varieties of his preferred foods without a problem," Ali shared with me.

Specifically, Ryder was continuing to eat strawberries and sweet potato fries. He was more consistently eating canned peaches, pears and macaroni and cheese and was welcoming cooked sweet potato in moderation. Just shy of twelve weeks into our time together, one of Ali's happiest developments was that Ryder was regularly eating grilled cheese cut into bite-size squares.

Of course, he still had room to grow, but Ryder's expanding diet demonstrated significant growth. He was now embracing more colorful and flavorful foods and more complex textures. From a practical standpoint, his nutritional intake had improved, and Ali felt more secure taking Ryder out to eat. In fact, she had gone to a restaurant with her family recently and ordered Ryder a grilled cheese with fries. She removed the crust from the grilled cheese, cut it into squares and almost cried when Ryder nonchalantly started eating without her assistance. To her surprise, Ryder also ate three bites of ravioli that her sister offered him. "It was a little dark and I think he didn't realize what it was at first," she said. "But he ate it!" It was clear that Ryder was beginning to trust himself with new foods and was learning to become a less cautious eater.

Ali had all the tools she needed to support Ryder in his journey to expand his diet. So, after about three and a half months, we put a pause on our regular sessions. When I checked in several weeks later, Ali only had good news to share. Ryder was continuing to eat more foods at school, and Ali was continuing to offer them at home. He was still tasting fruit more consistently, but vegetables remained a struggle. This, I assured Ali, was not something to be discouraged about. Vegetables are notoriously tricky for kids. They're not even most adults' favorite. Ryder's resistance to vegetables was more likely a symptom of typical toddler picky eating. His continuing to embrace new foods was a sign that he was overcoming the barriers that had interfered with his eating a diverse diet. Even without a variety of preferred vegetables, Ryder was continuing in the right direction.

Ryder's eating aptitude continued to grow. At a

different meal out, about eight weeks after Ali shared his last restaurant win, Ali went to help Ryder cut his grilled cheese and found him biting directly into the sandwich half, which he was holding in two hands! Ryder had previously never taken bites out of anything. He finished the whole sandwich as it was served, no cutting required. It was a lot of food for Ryder and a huge development.

With Ryder's sustained progress, Ali's anxiety began to subside. Optimism was finally overpowering her concern. She had come to realize that Ryder's eating journey would be an ongoing evolution. She accepted that he would continue to embrace new foods at his own pace and was now satisfied that his intake was adequate. While she might have to address Ryder's dietary habits for years, she was finally confident that he wasn't going to be stuck eating only a handful of foods forever. It no longer mattered to her whether Ryder's eating struggles were typical. She was now assured that they weren't permanent, and that was a more valuable takeaway than being able to pinpoint where he lay on the picky eating spectrum.

Activity: Building Food Bridges

Extremely picky kids eat the foods they do for a reason. Often these reasons are rooted in foods' sensory qualities. Many parents feel trapped by these restrictions, but I like to flip the perspective: Your child is clear about what they will eat, so take that and work with it!

Building food bridges is a tool to help identify and introduce new foods that your picky eater will be most likely to accept. A food bridge or chain originates with an accepted food, one that your child eats willingly and reliably, and ends with a number of novel foods. The chain is created by making gradual changes to the accepted food. As the chain grows, the foods become more and more diverse.

Bridging between preferred and novel foods is so effective for restrictive eaters because it takes into account the sensory experience of eating. It therefore minimizes the anxiety that many picky eaters feel when encountering new foods.

Building Bridges from Favorite Foods to Novel Ones

1. Create a list of all the foods that your child currently eats.

2. Identify any sensory qualities that the foods share. Consider the temperature, taste, texture, smell, shape and color. These are your child's preferences and the qualities you will use to help your child expand their diet.

3. Begin to build the bridge by introducing a new yet similar food that shares the preferred sensory qualities, but has one small yet significant change. Or, take a preferred

food and make a small change to its appearance, taste, temperature or texture. Start with almost imperceptible changes if your child is a more extreme picky eater. A less severe picky eater can tolerate more significant changes.

4. As your child comes to accept new foods, continue to introduce additional new items or incorporate new changes following the same principle. Aim to change just one sensory quality at a time and introduce a new food or new adjustments only when your child has regularly accepted the new food at least three times.

Sample Food Bridges/Food Chains

Chicken nuggets to baked fish

Chicken nuggets → fish nuggets (same look, similar taste) → fish sticks (same taste and texture, new look) → fish patty (same taste and texture, new look) → breaded fried white fish (similar taste, look and texture) → baked white fish

Veggie straws to veggies

Veggie straws → snap pea crisps (same texture and look) → freeze-dried green beans (similar look, similar texture) → raw green beans (same look, new texture) → raw asparagus (same look, new texture and taste) → lightly steamed asparagus (same look, new texture)

Potato chips to bananas

Potato chips → salted plantain chips (similar look and texture, new taste) → banana chips (same texture and look, new taste) → freeze-dried bananas (same look and taste) → frozen banana slices (same look, new texture) → fresh banana slices (same look, new texture)

Fries to carrots

French fries → sweet potato fries (same shape, new color and taste) → butternut squash fries (same shape and color, new taste) → roasted butternut squash cubes (same taste and color, new shape)→ roasted carrot cubes (same shape and color, new taste) → steamed carrots (same taste and color, new texture)

Applesauce to apples

Regular applesauce → natural sugar-free applesauce (same look and texture, similar taste) → chunky applesauce (same flavor, similar look, new texture) → homemade chunky applesauce (same look and texture, similar taste) → baked apple slices (same flavor, similar look, similar texture) → fresh apple slices (similar look, similar taste, new texture)

Peaches to pineapples

Sliced peaches → frozen sliced peaches (new texture, same look and taste) → frozen cubed peaches (same texture and taste, new look) → frozen pineapple (same shape and texture, new taste) → dried pineapple (similar look and taste, new texture) → fresh pineapple (same look and taste, new texture)

CHAPTER 4

Can I Get a Lunch Pass?

A Child Who Can't Eat at School

It wasn't until Charlie's eight-month-old sister began eating table food that Emily realized that Charlie was having a hard time. Charlie wasn't a bad eater, but there were two areas where he struggled with food. A common and relatively simple one to address was a resistance to trying new foods. Charlie refused to try any food that was not either chocolatey or already an established component of his limited diet. He had been limiting his range of accepted foods over the past two years, since he was about eighteen months old. Emily couldn't remember the last time he had welcomed anything new.

The second issue, the one that gnawed at Emily the most and that I quickly realized would be the more challenging habit to overcome, was that Charlie didn't eat a single thing—not even his most preferred foods—while he was at preschool.

At the time we started working together, Charlie, approaching four years old, was only in school for four hours a day two days a week. Emily knew that in the grand scheme of things, skipping lunch two days out of every seven was not the end of the world, so initially she brushed her concern aside. Yet, within the next few months, Charlie would be going to school for six hours a day five days a week. Emily's worry was beginning to build.

Charlie's not eating lunch didn't initially stand out to me as much as two other characteristics of his eating habits. First, Charlie favored foods picky eaters traditionally avoid. Eating even a single vegetable was rare for the extreme picky eaters I've encountered; however, Charlie's limited diet included a variety of them. Additionally, Charlie seemed to favor mixed dishes, sauces and even some bold flavors. The stereotypical picky eater likes plain: plain pasta, plain chicken, white bread with no crust. Yet Charlie loved chicken curry with rice and preferred spaghetti not dry but with meatballs, Bolognese sauce or carbonara sauce.

Second, though Charlie was not interested in consuming nonpreferred foods, he was interested in food in general. Emily told me that when sharing a meal with his parents and grandparents, Charlie was typically curious about what they were eating, commonly jutting his face close to their plates to examine the unfamiliar contents. His family was quick to offer him a taste, but Charlie always responded with a polite "No, thank you." I observed this during my sessions with Charlie and in recordings of his meals. He was curious to examine novel foods visually but held back when it came to touching or tasting them.

Emily ultimately had two goals for Charlie: She wanted him to eat at school and to broaden his diet so he could eat more family meals. I anticipated that we could work on each simultaneously, but I didn't expect the approach for each to be the same. I intended to uncover the root of Charlie's resistance to eating at school by learning more about the mealtime environment and examining what Emily had tried already.

As we worked to create a plan for Charlie's lunches, I'd

also be providing direction for the rest of his meals at home. From my discussions with Emily so far, I planned to address the mealtime environment before developing tactics that would inspire Charlie to try new foods. Overall, my goal was to gently push Charlie outside of his comfort zone, so he was eating more diversely both at home and at school.

For the sake of readability here, I'm going to first recap our experience working with Charlie's lunchtime struggles before reviewing the process I used to help Charlie try new foods.

When Emily first told me about Charlie and school, I figured there must be an obvious explanation. He wasn't the first child I'd encountered who opted out of school meals, so I wasn't even particularly concerned. Many kids struggle to concentrate and relax enough to eat sufficiently in the noisy shared spaces where lunchtime occurs. Some simply aren't hungry at the designated time. On top of that, others can't effectively open their lunch boxes, don't have enough time to eat or feel too anxious to be able to get something down.

After Charlie's first two weeks at school, Emily wasn't initially surprised to learn that he wasn't eating the school-provided lunch. In addition to his struggles eating novel foods, Charlie habitually wrestled with change, so Emily allowed him time to adapt to the new experience without worrying. But even after Charlie settled in, began to make friends and started to look forward to his days at school, he still didn't eat the lunch they served. Water was the only thing he consumed all day long.

Emily had tried a number of times to find out what was standing in Charlie's way and persuade him to eat lunch with his peers. When she couldn't identify a clear barrier, she began sending Charlie with a packed lunch of his most preferred foods, thinking his apprehension of the unfamiliar foods the school served was the problem. It didn't make a difference. After a few months, she was distraught and unsure of how to proceed.

In terms of interventions, Emily hadn't done much. Beyond talking with Charlie and sending him with lunch, she wasn't sure how to help him or even whether she needed to. She was constantly wondering whether his not eating would eventually resolve on its own.

Catching up on Charlie's lunch experience so far, I had the same questions Emily had. Was lunchtime too noisy? Too smelly? Was he even hungry? Did he have enough time? She had asked Charlie a number of times what the issue was. Each answer was a dead end. Charlie didn't endorse any of these issues, but Emily wasn't certain that he comprehended what she was asking. According to Charlie's teachers, lunchtime at school was comfortable and calm. They reported that Charlie never once complained or seemed to indicate any distress. If it wasn't for his not eating, he would have appeared entirely fine. After ruling out obvious sensory triggers in the lunch environment, I figured we'd start with a few small steps that could inspire Charlie to change his behavior.

I agreed that Emily should continue to pack Charlie's lunch. He didn't mind that he was the only one who brought a lunch to school, and, because his acceptance of novel foods was a work in progress, having his preferred foods to eat created one less barrier he had to overcome. During our first session, I presented Emily with an idea of how we could use Charlie's packed lunch to our advantage. Because hands-on experiences like cooking, gardening and food shopping are linked to increased likeliness of eating, I recommended that Emily include Charlie in selecting, preparing and packing his meal.[53,54,55,56]

Charlie welcomed the opportunity to help. He was used to serving as Emily's sous chef, so the kitchen was a familiar and comfortable space. The first time, he diligently selected items and arranged them in his lunch box. He picked the same foods that Emily usually packed and seemed to enjoy the responsibility of helping to make decisions that were usually reserved for his mom. "It was a really positive experience," Emily told me afterward, noting that Charlie had fun. Enjoyment is another factor associated with increased willingness to eat, so I was optimistic.[57] Unfortunately, Charlie's participation and enjoyment didn't translate to his lunch box coming home emptier. He still didn't eat.

Emily continued to include Charlie in packing his lunch. Just because it did not have an immediate effect on his eating, there was no guarantee that it never would. Plus, his time in the kitchen was still valuable in improving his general relationship with food.

Because, according to Emily, Charlie was a creature of habit, my next attempt, which we addressed a week later, was to create a connection between his eating environments at home and at school. My hope was that having something familiar from his home environment—a special cup, for example—at preschool would serve as a comfort that would both cue Charlie to eat and communicate to him that school was a safe and comfortable environment for him to do so. Emily thought this approach would work well, but Charlie didn't have a transferrable constant in his current mealtime routine, so instead of adapting something he was currently using, I suggested we create a new one. Charlie could start using it at home and then bring it to school, where I hoped it would serve as a cue to eat.

Charlie was immediately hooked on the plain blue place mat that Emily bought for him later that week. He proudly assumed the new role of setting his place at their dining table, and the place mat soon became something he didn't want to have a meal without. However, the place mat never made it to school. Emily suggested they pack it up a handful of mornings, but Charlie had become so attached to it that he didn't want to let it outside of the house. After two weeks of encouraging him to take the place mat to school, Emily stopped. We decided to revisit the issue and possibly purchase a second place mat if we failed to find another solution.

Next, I wanted to revisit the environmental aspects of school lunch. As far as we knew, Charlie didn't have sensory issues, but it was still possible that something modifiable was interfering with his desire to eat. We learned from Charlie's teachers that lunch started with handwashing. Then, the kids ate at the same tables in the same classroom where they conducted many of the day's other activities. According to Charlie's teachers, lunchtime was relatively quiet and calm, and Charlie seemed as comfortable during lunch as he did throughout the rest of the day.

Nothing stood out to us, but I still wondered if something in this seemingly benign process was rubbing Charlie the wrong way. Maybe he didn't like eating in front of others. Maybe he couldn't focus. I advised Emily to see if Charlie could eat in a quiet space on his own one day. His teachers, equally as concerned about Charlie's failure to eat, happily obliged. Yet Charlie, who loved eating one-on-one with his family members, still didn't eat in a private room alone with his teacher.

Throughout our time together, I had been relying on Emily for information about Charlie's school, as I had never visited. But it turned out, she hadn't either. Given that nothing so far had worked, I suggested Emily stop by during lunchtime one day. I thought it would be beneficial for her to observe Charlie and the environment for herself. I also wondered if maybe, like the place mat I was hoping Charlie would bring to school, she could actually be the trigger that Charlie needed to eat.

Emily called with both good and bad news as soon as she got home from Charlie's school that day. The good news: Although Charlie seemed quieter than usual during lunch, she confirmed that he was not uncomfortable, bothered or unsafe. The bad news: Even with Emily's company, gentle encouragement and her eating by his side, Charlie still did not eat.

Over the next several weeks that Emily and I continued to work together, Charlie made some small developments with his school lunches. According to his teachers, he began to interact more with his meal, opening his lunch box and touching his food—things he had never done before. These interactions mirrored ones that we had simultaneously been working on with Charlie at home. They represented progress but were not significant enough achievements to make us confident that he would be eating any time soon.

Emily and I were both anticipating the start of a new school year, when Charlie would be attending a new school five days a week, as a fresh opportunity. A fresh start with a different routine and environment might be what Charlie needed. The week before school started, Emily took Charlie shopping for a new lunch box. Charlie picked one that he liked, his casual, calm demeanor belying his yearlong struggle with the meal it contained. His ease at the store helped calm Emily, but it didn't resolve the questions she had: Would the lunch box make a difference? Would he use it? Should she even bother?

On the first day at his new school, Charlie willingly brought along his new lunch box packed with his favorite foods that he helped to select. Emily waited anxiously the whole day. When she finally picked him up, Charlie met her holding his heavy lunch box. He hadn't eaten.

Emily had remained positive and open-minded with each new attempt and subsequent disappointment. She tried all of my suggestions despite Charlie's lack of progress. She had been holding out for his transition to a new school. With another letdown, her concern and confusion were mounting. The situation didn't make sense. Charlie ate at birthday parties and on airplanes. What was it about school?

By this point, Charlie knew that Emily was worried. In addition to having asked Charlie a number of times about why he wasn't eating, every day when she picked him up, the first thing Emily did was peer inside his lunch box and ask whether he had eaten. Emily didn't think he was the kind of kid to act out for attention. In fact, Charlie didn't like when there was a big fuss made over him. I felt the increased focus on his eating over the past few weeks couldn't be helping his anxiety or the underlying issue and that Charlie might have been sensing an added pressure, which I felt would make things worse.

Given this, our failed attempts to find a resolution and the absence of a clear sense of what was standing in Charlie's way, I felt it was time to back off and see if he changed on his own. I advised Emily to proceed as if Charlie's lunchtime behavior was not an issue and to keep lunchtime talk to a minimum unless he brought it up. She should no longer ask Charlie whether he had eaten or was hungry when she picked him up from school. His teachers also didn't need to urge him to eat or make any special accommodations.

Food refusal is a normal part of development for young children. Saying "no" is an act of independence, a way for a young child to exercise their autonomy. Trying too hard to get Charlie to eat could translate to him rebelling at lunch or during his meals at home and could erode the trust he had in Emily as his caretaker.

We had done our best to make sure that there was no modifiable barrier that could make eating at school easier for Charlie, but in the end, it wasn't our job to get him to eat. Our job was to ensure he had a comfortable and positive eating environment at school and that he had a well-balanced meal that he was capable of eating. We had done that. Ultimately, we couldn't—and shouldn't—

force Charlie to eat at school. So, we moved forward with the hope and trust that this was just a phase and that he would eventually come around when left to his own devices.

While working to resolve Charlie's struggles eating at school, Emily and I were simultaneously addressing his resistance to trying new foods. Based on my early conversations with Emily, I had a good idea of what Charlie ate and how he struggled, but these details didn't give me clues on how I could best help him. So, my first objective was to obtain more information about Charlie's habits and his mealtime environment. Specifically, I wanted to learn how often he was eating, how long meals lasted, who he ate with, where he ate and how he behaved. Eating is, of course, about food, but details about intake, portions and preferences alone fail to capture the complexity of eating and the breadth of potential factors that might contribute to a child's inability to eat well.

Emily told me that Charlie tended to get bored while eating. He fidgeted at the table and had trouble staying focused for the duration of his meal. His behavior was disruptive enough that Emily sometimes fed him or let him play on a tablet while he ate, which helped him sit for much longer. Emily told me that she found it interesting that Charlie actually behaved and ate much better during his regular lunch dates at his grandmother's house. Emily thought the individual attention and mealtime chats with his grandmother must have been the reason for his improved attention. I had a different idea.

I noticed that at home, Charlie ate seated on a bench at the kitchen table. The table was a little high for him, so he often sat with his feet tucked under his bum. In videos of him eating, I noticed that he was frequently readjusting his position. For comparison, I asked Emily to share photos of Charlie eating at his grandma's. She sent me a picture of Charlie seated in an old highchair that had its tray removed, so the chair aligned flush with the table. The chair hugged him securely. He didn't have any room to wiggle around. "It's like his throne," Emily told me. "If you ask Charlie, that's the comfiest chair in the whole world."

A child's seat can have a tremendous impact on their ability to make it through a meal. When sitting is hard, eating is hard. When eating is too hard, kids simply don't do it. If a child is uncomfortable at the table or does not have the strength and endurance to consume a full meal, they may have trouble supporting themselves and may then struggle to chew and swallow appropriately, which makes them more likely to choke. Providing a child with a supportive seat can be a game changer, improving both fidgeting at the table and fussy eating.

The ideal eating position for kids and adults alike includes 90-degree support at the waist, knees and ankles. If a child's feet do not reach the ground, they might benefit from a footrest to provide further stabilization and prevent swaying. Often, a highchair or children's table offers an ideal setup that allows kids to preserve their attention for eating instead of focusing on keeping their bodies upright. This makes eating safer, less tiresome and more successful.

Charlie's old highchair appropriately supported him at his back and hips. It also had a little shelf where he could rest his feet while eating. When sitting, his hips, knees and feet were all at 90-degree angles. Given how supportive this chair was, I wasn't surprised that he ate so well when seated there. Unfortunately, the bench at home wasn't giving him what he needed.

Emily invested in a booster seat that she could latch onto the bench where Charlie usually ate and created a makeshift footrest out of a cardboard box, so his feet didn't dangle. The booster supported him and also elevated his body, so he had a better position at the table. Emily realized that Charlie could also sit at the kid-sized table he usually used for crafts. Without any adjustments, it was the perfect setup for him.

I warned Emily that fixing Charlie's chair likely wasn't going to cure his aversion to new foods. Adjusting the chair had the explicit intent of making it easier, safer and more comfortable for him to eat. I also anticipated that sitting with the proper support would improve his attention span and minimize the need for assistance or distractions at mealtimes.

The adjustments seemed to do the trick for Charlie's ability to focus. Immediately, he was less fidgety during meals at home and was no longer inclined to get up from the table. It was hard to say what if any direct effect the modifications had on his eating because at the same time, we introduced additional mealtime adjustments that would help him expand his diet and improve his relationship with food.

With the simple adjustment to Charlie's physical environment at mealtimes out of the way, I next wanted to address several other details about how his mealtimes occurred. From one of our early discussions I learned that Emily was making him his own special meals, that he was often eating on his own and that she was not regularly serving him new foods. These habits were efficient and practical, but they were not providing Charlie with the exposures or opportunities he needed to step outside of his comfort zone. Additionally, they were adding to Emily's stress about Charlie's eating. Therefore, my next attempt to support Charlie in trying new foods would focus on helping Emily institute shared family meals where Charlie would naturally be encountering new foods daily.

Emily had been feeling overwhelmed making multiple meals for her family. Every night she diligently prepared a meal for her and her husband, made a variety of nutritious selections for her daughter and resorted to making Charlie either spaghetti with a sauce, fish sticks or chicken curry. In addition, Emily had gotten into the habit of asking Charlie what he wanted each night. He usually had an answer for her, and she accommodated it, finding that he ate better when she gave him exactly what he requested.

Emily might have been promoting Charlie's intake in the short term, but she wasn't doing his diet any favors in the long run. By allowing him to dictate his dinner menu, she was ensuring that he only encountered familiar foods and was actually reinforcing the selective eating habits that she was seeking to improve. Providing special meals to a selective eater does not foster an open-minded appetite or encourage the development of new food preferences. Instead, it reinforces a child's notion that they have their own special food and don't eat what everyone else does. On top of that, as Emily already knew, making multiple meals was a lot of work. Her ultimate goal was to serve one meal for her whole family. There was no reason she couldn't begin doing so now.

At first, Emily couldn't wrap her head around the adjustment. She wanted to expose her daughter to as many foods as possible, and Charlie needed to eat, which meant he had to have his preferred foods. She worried that she'd have to compromise if she only made one meal. Charlie's sister was mostly able to eat the foods that Emily and her husband did, but unless she served spaghetti, fish sticks or curry every night, Emily didn't see an easy way to accommodate everyone's preferences. I agreed that she shouldn't compromise on the quality and diversity of her daughter's diet simply because her son didn't like new foods. I could help her figure out how to devise a single menu that would expose Charlie to new foods, incorporate his preferred ones and continue to develop her daughter's diet.

To do so, I recommended that Emily plan one meal for herself, her husband and her daughter. All she had to do for Charlie was incorporate at least one food that he consistently ate. So, Emily could prepare pizza or grilled fish with salad and roasted potatoes, two meals that she made weekly for herself and her husband, and supplement with a side of spaghetti or Charlie's favorite vegetables.

Ensuring that a selective eater can come to the table and see something that they're comfortable with allows them to feel secure, which is extremely important, especially when implementing changes to the mealtime routine and gently pushing a picky eater outside of their comfort zone. The presence of a preferred food on the table communicates to the child that they are being cared for and lets them know that they won't sit down to an unmanageable experience or leave the meal hungry. However, with the purposeful lack of multiple preferred items, this style of meal also creates space for a selective eater to consider eating something they might not otherwise try and sends the message that they are capable of eating novel foods.

Of course, Emily could provide more than one of Charlie's preferred foods. She could even serve his preferred foods as the shared main. As long as there was something on the table that everyone liked to eat, she was doing her job. It was then up to Charlie to decide whether he wanted to eat and how much of each item he wanted to eat.

This principle—that parents and children have unique roles at the dinner table—forms the basis of Ellyn Satter's Division of Responsibility for Feeding. The Division of Responsibility is based on the idea that when parents dictate what is served and children manage whether and what they eat at mealtimes, everyone is less stressed and children are more likely to become more confident, flexible eaters.[58]

Serving one family meal didn't mean that Emily couldn't still welcome Charlie's input. I encouraged her to continue inviting his opinion on meal plans, but I asked her to revise her approach. Participation in food-related decisions and activities positively impacts a child's eating. It's when a child has *too much* say that the dynamic becomes unproductive.

I suggested that Emily avoid asking Charlie the general "What do you want for dinner?" question. Instead, she could present him with two nutritionally equivalent alternatives, which is just enough choice to foster a sense of control but not enough to present an overwhelming decision. For example: "Would you like pasta or potatoes, grapes or berries, apple in slices or chunks?" These simple selections keep menu planning within the caregiver's domain and ensure that the answer is one they're happy to hear. Just as importantly, it involves the child in an easy way that can be meaningful enough to increase their inclination to eat. This technique can be just as effective for preferred foods as it is for novel ones. I warned her that Charlie might at times proclaim that he wanted neither alternative. I recommended that if that happened, she should remind him that this was his opportunity to have a say in what he ate. One of the foods would end up on the table, so if Charlie had a preference, he should share it or Emily would decide.

With Emily finally preparing one meal, we turned our attention to working on the family eating together all at once. As things were, the family was not in the habit of sharing meals. Emily was on board with changing this. She loved the idea of spending less time in the kitchen and more time enjoying her family. She designated several times during the week, including breakfasts and lunches, when at least one parent could eat with Charlie and his sister. My express intention of recommending family meals was to give Charlie the opportunity to see his family eating foods he would be learning to taste, but he was bound to enjoy additional benefits. Kids who regularly share family meals eat more vegetables, demonstrate closer family relationships and have enhanced communication, empathy and emotional intelligence.[59]

Emily began serving shared meals with a single menu immediately following our second session together. Within two weeks, twice weekly dinners and the occasional breakfast or lunch had become their new norm. Charlie embraced their new mealtime routine. As usual, he enjoyed surveying what his parents were eating. In video clips of his mealtimes, I saw Charlie sitting comfortably eating his preferred foods while his parents and sister ate theirs. As usual, he asked questions about his family's food and, as usual, he declined when they offered him a bite.

Although Charlie enjoyed eating with his family, he didn't immediately come to enjoy eating their foods. He continued to eat his safe foods only, but observing his parents and sister easily eat and engage with their own meals was still a valuable experience for him. The sensory exposure—hearing the sounds of eating, smelling the smells and seeing what it all looked like—was helping to build his comfort with new foods, and, importantly, his family's enjoyment of their meal was something he was also registering. Although he wasn't yet ready to eat the foods he witnessed his family eating, their behavior was certainly providing an example that would eventually pay off.

I had already warned Emily to expect that Charlie likely would not eat new foods immediately. If he wasn't interested in the family's meal, he could stick with his preferred food. Emily always could—and should—offer the other foods, but she should respect his decision. Still, I didn't anticipate that Charlie would initiate eating novel foods on his own. Therefore, our next step was to address how to nudge Charlie closer to eating his family's novel foods. What should Emily do when Charlie repeatedly ignored all of the other food on the table? I scheduled our next session for just a week later to answer this question.

Emily was in the habit of pre-plating meals. Most of the serving dishes remained in the kitchen, and she brought prepared plates to the table. I asked if instead she would be open to serving family style, bringing all the food to the table in shared serving dishes and serving there. In their current routine, Emily was largely making assumptions about what and how much Charlie would eat. Moreover, without the serving dishes on the table, it didn't even seem like the family's food was intended for Charlie. Family-style serving would reinforce the concept that the family food was intended for everyone.

While these were meaningful details and ones that would help Charlie learn to eat new foods, the primary reason I wanted Emily to try family-style serving was because I wanted Charlie to serve himself. Family-style meals invite a sense of agency that children find very motivating. Instead of passively accepting a plate, they can dictate how much they'd like to take. If a child is not ready to welcome a food, they can opt to pass the dish. However, even simply passing a serving dish creates a natural interaction with novel foods. In doing so, a child is bringing the food into their personal space. They might smell it. They'll probably look at it. These incidental exposures form the foundation that children require to build their comfort eating new foods.

Emily was on board with one small hesitation. Wouldn't serving meals family style create more work and dishes to wash after each meal? In a brainstorming session, we came up with the idea to serve dishes in the pots or pans they were cooked in or the containers that they would eventually be stored in. Problem solved!

Charlie was eager to participate in the adult world. He seemed to take pride in passing the dishes that weren't too heavy for him to hold, and he appreciated the opportunity to inspect the food that went by. For the first few meals, we permitted Charlie to serve himself only the foods that he wanted and bypass anything outside of his comfort zone. Left on his own, he opted, unsurprisingly, to do exactly that. This was fine for the first few meals as Charlie was adapting to the new eating routine, but I soon wanted to actually get some novel foods on his plate. Welcoming even just a teeny spoonful of a new food in front of him would begin to prep him for eventually eating something new. Although it had only been two weeks, Charlie wasn't yet showing any inclination that he was ready to serve himself even the smallest portion of a new food, and we didn't foresee him changing any time soon. Emily and I agreed to meet a week later to discuss how we could encourage Charlie to interact more with novel and nonpreferred meals.

Although we knew Charlie wasn't averse to being close to nonpreferred foods, we weren't sure how he'd respond to having them on his plate during mealtimes. Rather than test the issue and risk completely alienating him, we decided to ease Charlie into increasingly intimate interactions with less familiar foods. To start this off, I advised Emily to set an extra plate on the table at Charlie's next meal. From now on, Charlie and his parents would serve themselves at least a tiny portion of every food that was on the dinner table. While they were always welcome to try something new, there was absolutely no requirement to eat every part of the meal. In fact, if they weren't even yet ready to welcome the new food on their dinner plate, they could place it on the extra plate, called the Exploring Plate.

The Exploring Plate was named for a reason. Eaters had to explore the foods that they placed there. For example, they could discuss the food's visual qualities or explore how it felt or tasted by squishing it, licking it or even taking a bite. The level of engagement could be as big or small as each individual desired. There would be no forcing Charlie to interact in a way that he wasn't yet comfortable with. My intention was to use the plate as a way to facilitate Charlie's working through Toomey's Steps to Eating. Whatever interaction he selected would build on his current comfort level and would therefore be a meaningful step in the right direction.

I encouraged Emily to include the Exploring Plate at all meals, even when Charlie was eating with just his sister, so he could engage with new foods daily. When they ate as a family, I suggested Charlie's parents participate in the Exploring Plate activities alongside him to ensure that he wouldn't feel singled out or like the task was a punishment. Instead, I hoped that the Exploring Plate would be welcomed as a fun opportunity that capitalized on his innate curiosity about food.

Charlie welcomed the Exploring Plate with ease and interest. Emily shared a video of the first night they used it. I watched as Charlie's dad placed a carrot, one of Charlie's preferred foods, on the plate. Emily was interested in a piece of chicken sausage and decided that she was comfortable placing it on her dinner plate with her meal. Charlie also selected a small piece of chicken sausage. He added it to the Exploring Plate alongside his father's carrot.

The family went about eating their dinner, Charlie sticking with spaghetti and safe vegetables. His parents and sister were enjoying chicken sausage with pesto sauce, roasted vegetables and pita bread. They also had small portions of Charlie's pasta on their plates. Midway through the meal, Emily initiated the exploring activity. She picked up her piece of chicken sausage and smelled it. "I smell lots of herbs, and there's a meaty smell, too," she said. Charlie's dad followed. He started mashing the carrot with his fork. "It's soft," he noticed. Then he took a bite. "It's sweet and a little salty. It's soft and easy to chew. Yum!" It was Charlie's turn. He looked to the Exploring Plate with some hesitation. "You can tell us what it looks like, Charlie," Emily prompted.

When I gave examples of interactions the family could use to explore new foods, Emily and I had discussed prompting Charlie using "can" phrases. Whereas questions and requests like "just try a bite" and "take a taste for me" can create pressure and expectation, "can" phrases create possibility and could actually empower Charlie. They would be effective at providing guidance and direction when Charlie stagnated. Once he had the idea, he could ultimately decide to act or not act in any way that he pleased.

Upon Emily's suggestion, Charlie described the sausage slice: sort of round and big. Because Charlie did well, Emily suggested he go a step further. "You can pick it up if you like," she offered. He did. Seeing that Charlie was comfortable with the tactile experience, Emily kept going: "You can lick it." As he did, Charlie's eyes went wide, and he made a face as if he was unsure of how to process the experience he'd just had. Sensing that he'd had enough, Emily complimented his achievement. Charlie looked pleased. He put the sausage down, but instead of returning it to the Exploring Plate, he placed it on his own.

Moving forward, every meal included a novel food that Charlie was encouraged to have an intentional interaction with. With increasing practice and exposure, he began to overcome his trepidation. After Emily had suggested it a few times, Charlie began to lick just about anything without hesitation. His grandparents were especially impressed when, during a family meal at their house within a week of Emily's introducing the Exploring Plate, Charlie picked up and repeatedly licked a piece of steak from a small portion he had beside him. Charlie enjoyed the positive feedback he got from his new accomplishment and didn't seem to experience any discomfort or anxiety from these more involved interactions.

I was really proud of Charlie and his apparent comfort experiencing new flavors and having unfamiliar foods near his face. Given the pace and ease of his progress, in our next session I suggested Emily encourage Charlie to move further along the Steps to Eating. For example, she could suggest that after licking, he could hold food on his tongue for a few seconds or take a tiny bite and chew a few times before either spitting the food out or even swallowing if he was ready.

Less than a week later, Emily reported that the new prompts were working. "I bought breaded chicken and Charlie spat out the first two mouthfuls, but then ate the rest!" she shared. That wasn't all. "Then last night we used the 'you can take a bite and spit it out,' and he did that with baby corn, sugar snap peas and a lemon and herb chicken breast that I had made. That seems to have been a really big step in him thinking, 'Well, I can just spit it out if I don't like it,' so he's more likely to have a bite!"

Charlie hadn't tried tasting something new in years, so this was a big deal for them both. I advised Emily to continue serving the breaded chicken as well as the corn, snap peas and chicken breast. The more Charlie encountered them, the more his comfort with them would grow and the more he would be inclined to permanently welcome them into his diet.

Even though Charlie was making impressive progress with tasting new foods, his core diet remained unchanged. Because his preferences were so limited, he was regularly eating the same foods several days in a row. Emily was often making spaghetti three days in a row, and Charlie's preferred vegetables made daily appearances. I worried it would be more challenging for him to embrace new foods if he encountered the same few foods prepared in the exact same way day after day. If variety became

Charlie's new norm, he would adapt and would eventually be more open to accepting new foods. Additionally, I wanted to preserve the foods that he liked. More diversity in his diet would limit his chances of first tiring of and then dropping them. Therefore, at our next session, Emily and I spoke about ways she could ensure that Charlie was not eating the same foods twice in one day or two days in a row.

In addition to creating a rotating menu, I recommended that Emily introduce slight modifications to Charlie's staples. For example, I suggested exploring new pasta shapes as well as different preparations and presentations of Charlie's preferred vegetables. Currently, Charlie ate broccoli, carrots and green beans prepared only one way. Emily could cut them differently or mix them together in unique combinations. These changes could be enough to minimize the risk of repetition while also priming Charlie to be less rigid with his food preferences.

"We've had some small wins," Emily said after she tried this new strategy for a few days. She served Charlie bow ties with carbonara sauce instead of spaghetti and broccolini in place of his usual broccoli. He ate them both. It had been a long time since Emily had veered from Charlie's staples. From her previous attempts at doing so, she never would have imagined that introducing something new could be that easy.

Charlie was demonstrating an increased openness and flexibility with his diet. I was confident that he was not destined to be a fussy eater forever. Still, like most children with feeding problems, sometimes Charlie would hear about the dinner menu or encounter a new dish and instinctively announce, "I don't like that." Emily felt defeated every time she heard him say this. She knew Charlie's declaration was inaccurate, but she wasn't sure how to help him realize this. Sometimes she ignored it. Sometimes she countered that Charlie couldn't possibly know what he liked and didn't like without trying it.

Emily and I were working hard to help Charlie see that he actually did like more than he thought, that he was the kind of kid who could eat all sorts of foods. So, I recommended she reply, "You don't like it *yet*," or, "You're still learning to like it," to reinforce to Charlie that his preferences might need time to develop. The importance of repeated exposures to new foods is something I share with all parents I work with. Emily was already familiar with the path that Charlie needed to embark on in order to establish his eating preferences, but Charlie was not. As soon as Emily shared Charlie's "I don't like it" behavior with me, I made time for him to join us in our next session.

Charlie was young, but he was intelligent. He enjoyed learning about how things worked and why things were the way they were. So, I sought to teach him about taste and how it develops. I described the experiments scientists had conducted to learn more about how kids grow to like different foods and flavors. I told Charlie that they found that sometimes we like the taste of a new food right away, but more often, we ultimately learn to like an unfamiliar food after we've tried it at least ten, and sometimes many more, times. I shared that when I was a little girl, I didn't like raw carrots or chocolate. (He couldn't believe that there was a child who didn't like chocolate.) My mom served carrots all the time and, well, chocolate was unavoidable. Because I kept encountering these foods, I kept trying them. "And guess what?" I asked. "Now I love chocolate, and I love carrots. I eat them almost every day. After multiple exposures, my body learned to like these delicious foods."

Charlie took this in with a nod. "You can learn to like new foods, too," I told him. "But you have to try them." It was Emily's duty to remind him of this whenever he dismissed a food before trying it. Charlie still didn't have to try a new food if he wasn't yet ready, but I wanted him to be open to the idea that he could learn to like new flavors and that he was a child who could enjoy a diverse diet.

Charlie's "I don't like it" reflex didn't disappear. He continued to instinctively respond this way when he was intimidated by a new food. The difference was that Emily now had a plan for how to effectively respond so that she was encouraging his growth. Charlie also had context about how his relationship with new foods would evolve.

Emily and I had been meeting for a little over three months when we decided to put our sessions on hold. Charlie was making great progress at home. He was continuing to expand his diet outside of mealtimes, constantly surprising Emily with his newfound flexibility and openness to novel foods. She told me a story that she found particularly promising. Charlie frequented a local café with his grandparents and always ordered white toast. One day, well into our time together, the café ran out of white bread and sent brown instead. Months ago, Charlie would have asked questions about it, but wouldn't have eaten it. However, on that day, he picked up the toast, licked it and then started to eat. He also told his grandparents that if they weren't ready to eat the toast yet, they could lick it first.

While Charlie wasn't that welcoming of every food he met, the toast experience wasn't an anomaly. He was becoming more open to trying new foods. Emily was also settling into their new normal. She had the tactics she needed to support Charlie's eating journey. Now, it was just a matter of time.

Around four months after our sessions had ended, I checked in with Emily. Charlie was continuing to gain confidence with new foods at home. He was touching, licking and trying more, and more importantly, he was discovering ones that he actually liked. He was finally beginning to expand his diet in a meaningful way.

Emily shared that she was still in search of a permanent

solution for Charlie's aversion to eating at school; however, Charlie actually had made some progress. Emily stayed for lunch one day after dropping Charlie off from an appointment. To her complete shock, Charlie ate in his classroom with her by his side, and he continued to do so—only if she was there—for an entire month. As soon as she stopped attending, he didn't eat. Something about Emily's presence helped Charlie eat, but she wasn't sure what it was or how to move forward. She was in the process of creating a long-term plan with a child psychologist who suspected that Charlie had sensory issues and, more importantly, anxiety that was holding him back from eating comfortably.

Despite the news about Charlie's anxiety and sensory impairments, this was the best update that I had received from Emily in several months. They were making progress. I was proud that Charlie was finally eating and just as proud of Emily for seeking and finally finding the help that he needed to further develop his ability to eat at school. Most importantly, I was now confident that Charlie would learn to comfortably eat lunch just as he had learned to comfortably try new foods.

Charlie was an example in so many ways of how the path to picky eating resolutions is rarely straightforward and rarely unfolds as we expect. His ability to finally eat at school may have been a combination of time and patience. It's just as likely that the progress he had made tasting and discovering new foods outside of the classroom contributed to his change in behavior. Ultimately, the combination of factors didn't matter. The only thing that mattered was that Charlie was having an easier time with eating. His intake at home had significantly improved, and a permanent solution for his eating at school was not far behind.

Activity: Food for Fun

If we can get kids touching their food, they'll be more likely to eat. Touching leads to learning how food feels, smells and behaves. This information makes kids feel safer tasting because they know what to expect. The only trouble is that skeptical eaters don't readily touch new foods! That's where food play comes in.

Playing with food is actually good for kids, and beyond that, it's a fun, low-pressure way for them to learn about and become more comfortable with new foods.

I know this sounds like a lot of work and mess. It can be both. But it's also one of the best things that you can do to encourage a fussy eater to expand their diet. Children who have positive hands-on experiences playing with food are more likely to try new food and eat a more varied diet. Plus, studies show that kids who play with their food have a greater vocabulary to talk about food.

Try to retrain your thinking. Mess is good. It's a sign your child is exploring and learning to become more comfortable with food. I assure you it's also usually not as bad as you think it will be. If you're concerned about cleanup, set them up over newspaper or a tarp. I like to line the play area in silicone place mats that are inexpensive, indestructible and easy to clean. I also recommend designating a smock or shirt for food play, especially if you're playing with purees or stainable foods, so you don't have to worry about ruined clothing.

Try these ideas to add food play outside of mealtimes:

Edible Collage: Grab a plate, a place mat or an area of a clean table. Using foods from a meal or a collection of new and familiar foods, create faces, animals, people, cars, flowers, houses or whatever scene your child wants. Incorporate dips or props and get creative with your materials.

Olives and beans make great eyes. Broccoli is a natural tree. Cheese or shredded chicken can become hair. You can even use a piece of food as your canvas. A halved baked potato or slice of bread with a spread works well.

Tic-Tac-Toe: Create a tic-tac-toe board using string beans or asparagus. You might need to line up a few to make it large enough, or you can make an extra big board for a more challenging game. Strips of bread and cheese also work well. Use a novel food as your game piece and get playing. It's okay to eat some of your pieces.

Munchable Masterpieces: Create structures using a variety of foods. Use sturdy foods like carrot sticks, chicken nuggets and crackers. String soft pierceable foods (pasta, banana slices, berries, meatballs, etc.) along a sturdy stick-shaped food like a raw vegetable or pretzel to make patterns or use the soft foods as corners to hold the pieces together. Anything works! Kids love the idea of using food to build, and it's always exciting to see how tall your tower can climb.

You can think of your own play schemes that incorporate your child's interests and can also try the simple activities below during a meal.

To encourage touching and smelling:
- Pretend a goal food is a train and use another food to push it along the tracks.
- Play peek-a-boo by hiding the goal food under a napkin.
- Create a bouquet by wrapping the goal food in a napkin; smell the flower.
- Smoosh a food with one finger or with the whole hand.
- Play hot potato.
- Line up foods in a size order.
- Pretend the goal food is a baby: cradle it in your

arms and kiss it goodnight before tucking it into bed (a napkin).

- Use long stick-like foods as drumsticks or magic wands.
- Paint with a sauce, puree or dip.
- Roll round foods around like wheels.
- Pretend the goal food is a mustache, beard, necklace, watch or bracelet.
- "Drive" a food up your arm and sit it on your shoulder. Say, "Look! I can drive my car up the mountain to the station!"
- Play telephone with the goal food.
- Build a tower.
- Use small cookie cutters to make shapes out of food.
- Pretend the food is a kangaroo that jumps on your head and shoulders.
- Put on makeup or shave using a puree.
- Break up pieces of the food to count or line up.
- Make a full handprint in a puree.
- Use purees as body paint to draw tattoos.

To encourage tasting:
- Hold a long stick-like food between your teeth like a dog with a bone.
- Create bite art using your teeth.
- Chew like different animals. Try a dinosaur, a bunny, a horse.
- Hold the food using only your teeth, with no hands.
- Play hide-and-seek in your mouth.
- Balance a food on the tip of your tongue.
- Take a quick taste like a snake, darting your tongue quickly in and out.

- Hold a food to your lips and blow it like a horn.
- Lick the food like a lollipop.
- Crunch a food so loud the neighbors can hear.
- Lick a food like a dog.
- "Brush your teeth" with a long stick-like food.
- Break a food into small pieces, hold them between your teeth or lips and blow them into a cup like basketball.
- Use only your tongue or lips to pick up a food from the table.
- Have a contest: see who can crunch a food the loudest using the back molars.

CHAPTER 5

Pizza Party

A Child Who Eats Pizza for Dinner Every Night

Abby's concern started rising when she noticed that most of her son's peers were outgrowing their picky eating habits, but his was just getting worse. Within recent months, Ryan had begun to shun the few healthier items in his diet, relying more on the sugar-rich processed snacks that Abby was perennially trying to phase out.

At five years old, Ryan was essentially eating four types of foods: starches, dairy products, packaged snacks and sweets. He had recently dropped his only three protein-rich options and was down to only a few nutritionally substantial alternatives. Peanut butter was still in favor and he ate it almost daily. Other than that, the bulk of his protein calories came from pizza, cereal, waffles and the increasingly rare grilled cheese.

Similarly, Ryan's fruit intake had recently dwindled; he was eating only raisins when I first met him. Abby rejoiced on the rare occasions that he accepted a fruit and vegetable puree pouch and was in constant shock that he gobbled up her homemade muffins, which were fortified with spinach or carrots, yogurt and oatmeal.

Really, though, Ryan could live on pizza alone. He ate

it every single evening. Abby had a freezer full of individual slices she stockpiled from his favorite restaurant. Ever since he began limiting his diet, it was one of the few things he consistently ate for dinner and the only item he ever asked for.

Abby wasn't only bothered that Ryan was getting pickier. She was also concerned about what his doing so meant for his nutritional well-being. Ryan was more of a grazer, and his intake at most meals seemed low to Abby. He didn't eat lunch most days, and even when he was hungry at dinner, he rarely finished his plate. Due to his decreased intake and slimmed-down list of preferred foods, he was consequently consuming more pizza and more high-sugar packaged snacks.

When Abby first approached me for support, she requested a list of healthier snack food ideas. She thought this would alleviate much of her stress. She reasoned that if the foods Ryan was eating were better, she wouldn't worry as much. While this is a common request, I knew that a list wouldn't give Abby the results she wanted—or likely any at all. We needed to address the root of Ryan's eating difficulties.

As Abby ran me through the details of Ryan's eating struggles—his frequent snacking, dwindling diet, insistence on pizza, poor intake at mealtimes and avoidance of new foods—and described his daily diet, I identified a more productive focus. First, Ryan didn't seem to be encountering new foods. Second, his eating schedule was off and was likely contributing to his poor intake at meals. If we could optimize these two areas, I was confident that Ryan's intake and preferences would both improve to the point where Abby no longer felt like she needed an index of foods to tempt him with.

I began our first full session discussing dinner, which was where Ryan's diet and intake were most limited and where

Abby was therefore struggling the most. Ryan's intake throughout the day was sporadic. After his morning snack at school, Ryan, apparently not hungry, refused the lunch that Abby packed him. Not long after, he usually had pretzels on his way to afternoon swimming lessons or behavioral therapy sessions, which he was attending for a possible spectrum disorder. He closed out the afternoon with another snack, again pretzels or a granola bar, in the car on the way home from those activities just before dinner. These mini meals temporarily tamed Ryan's hunger yet failed to actually keep him full. Most evenings, he walked in the door famished, demanding dinner immediately. These were the times that he insisted on having pizza, often going into the freezer himself to get it.

Even though Ryan's focus on pizza didn't sit well with her, Abby didn't discourage Ryan's behavior. She always gave him what he wanted. In fact, she admitted that she actually considered Ryan's insistence to be an opportunity. After a day of lackluster intake, she thought she should take advantage of his hunger by providing the one meal he was guaranteed to eat.

Additionally, Abby was proud of Ryan for letting her know that he was hungry. Ryan had expressive language delay. At five, he lacked a vigorous vocabulary and was not always able to verbalize his needs and desires. Abby was compelled to reward him when he communicated effectively, and she worried that disregarding his request for pizza could deter him from voicing desires in the future.

Furthermore, though Ryan had never been a skinny kid or had any concerning health issues or problems with his growth, Abby worried about his nutritional well-being. She knew that abstaining from one of the day's three major meals meant Ryan likely wasn't acquiring all of the nutrition that his body needed, especially because he compensated with junk food. So, whenever he expressed interest in eating at night, she jumped at the opportunity. When Ryan said, "This is what I want," she happily obliged.

Yet even when Abby served Ryan, who was apparently hungry, a half slice of pizza with a side of raisins—two of his favorite foods and exactly what he'd indicated he wanted—he rarely ate a substantial portion. Based on a food diary that Abby completed and shared with me before our sessions, Ryan always left food on his plate. Because of this, Abby struggled with what meals would actually look like if she didn't serve pizza every night. Ryan ate so few foods. What else could she offer that he would actually eat?

Before addressing Abby's question about what to serve for dinner, I wanted to first absolve her of one of her major sources of stress. Abby needed to stop fixating on how much Ryan ate. I understood the source of Abby's concern and I agreed that Ryan's intake had room for improvement. However, worrying or attempting to micromanage his diet wouldn't help. In fact, both would likely make Ryan's eating worse.

Abby wanted Ryan to grow up having a healthy relationship with food. She knew too well how the ramifications of feeling pressured to eat as a child could extend to adulthood. She wanted her son to grow up knowing how to comfortably and confidently eat what he needed. I explained that her interfering with his natural inclinations to eat by pressuring, catering to his desires or even continuing to suggest that Ryan have his leftovers before bed could backfire. I told her about Ellyn Satter's Division of Responsibility for Feeding, which is founded in the belief of a child's inherent capacity to trust their own hunger and fullness cues. Ryan, who was comfortable leaving food on his plate, already seemed tuned into his body's needs. Abby needed to start trusting them, too.

I explained to Abby that in order for Ryan to expand his diet, she needed to stop obsessing about how much he ate. Ryan's eating would only improve if they shared a mutual trust when it came to his eating. I believed that feeding him would be much easier for Abby if she trusted that he was responding to his hunger cues. Importantly, once she did, she could stop catering to his demands and begin to introduce Ryan to a more nutritious diet.

The other side of this was Ryan's learning to understand that while he might not always get pizza for dinner, he could still rely on Abby's serving him consistent and appropriate meals. That is exactly what Abby and I discussed next.

At the time we met, Abby's primary focus at dinnertime was respecting Ryan's preferences and getting the meal on the table as quickly as possible before he decompensated. In her mind, pizza seemed to be not just the easiest option, but the only one. She didn't have a single idea when I asked her for possible alternatives. Although pizza was Ryan's favorite, when I reviewed his list of preferred foods, I saw that it wasn't the only dinner-appropriate food that he ate. His peanut butter sandwiches, her homemade muffins and even guacamole and chips could serve as dinner options.

I asked Abby if she had ever considered planning Ryan's menu in advance. That way, she wouldn't have to come up with meals on the fly. Abby couldn't believe she hadn't thought of the idea on her own. She told me that she regularly menu planned for her own meals with her husband. How had she never thought about it for the kids? We discussed the many benefits. If Abby created the menu and shared it with Ryan in advance, it would help him learn not to expect pizza every night. Additionally, Abby wouldn't be as inclined to give in to his demands. Ryan would love it, she told me. She described her son as particular and rigid. He liked consistency and knowing what to expect. A planned menu, she felt, was just what he needed.

Because Abby had trouble envisioning a week's worth of varied meals for Ryan, we compiled a master list of foods that she could use to create his weekly menu. It included preferred foods that were appropriate for dinner, foods that Ryan used to eat and, because Ryan loved dips, favorite condiments to add more variety to frequently repeated meals.

Ryan's Preferred Dinner Foods
- Pizza
- Grilled cheese (sometimes)
- Peanut butter sandwich
- French fries (frozen and from restaurants)
- Waffles with peanut butter
- Abby's homemade muffins
- Guacamole and chips (sometimes)
- Hummus and chips (sometimes)

Foods Ryan Used to Eat
- Grapes
- Raspberries
- Strawberries
- Pineapple chunks
- Apples, whole
- Chicken nuggets
- Rigatoni with pureed meat sauce

Ryan's Preferred Dips
- Ketchup
- Cheese sauce
- Maple syrup
- Jam
- Honey
- Vanilla icing
- Butter

I recommended that Abby plan to include one or two preferred items, which we defined as foods that Ryan ate more than 50 percent of the times he was offered them, at every meal. Additionally, once Ryan adapted to the menu concept, I encouraged her to routinely incorporate one new or formerly preferred food with meals. My intention was not just to wean Ryan from his nightly pizza party and ensure that Abby had enough pizza-free alternatives; I was also preparing Ryan to expand his diet. With this framework in mind, Abby and I began planning out a few meals that included at least one filling preferred food supplemented with a side of a less preferred food. One option was a peanut butter sandwich with an apple. Alternatively, she could try hummus with chips, cheese sauce and a muffin.

Once I shared these concrete ideas of how to plan the menu, which she agreed seemed workable, Abby introduced some of her own ideas on how to make it even more effective. Because of his language delay, Ryan was used to relying on pictures as guides. So, Abby decided she would create the menu using pictures, which would allow Ryan to easily understand what to expect for the upcoming week. Additionally, Abby thought to introduce theme nights, like Pizza Fridays and grilled cheese after swim lessons, as one extra way to reinforce routine and Ryan's expectations. I loved these ideas and for the first time in a long time, Abby was excited to feed her son.

When Abby and I touched base for a check-in a little over a week later, weaning off of pizza and sticking to a set menu were still works in progress. Abby told me that Ryan refused grilled cheese on two different nights, and when he asked for pizza instead, she gave in. She felt she was getting more resolute, but admitted that she struggled to deny him when he made a specific request.

I didn't want Ryan to feel that Abby wasn't considering his preferences at mealtimes, but if he continued to dictate the menu, pizza would remain a mainstay and Abby's frustration would grow. So, before going into our next plan, I gave Abby a few scripts to try that acknowledged Ryan's requests without capitulating to his demands. When he refused to eat, she could say: "Not every meal will be your favorite, but you can still eat." When he requested pizza, she could try: "I understand that you're hungry and I know you love pizza. This is what's on the menu tonight. Look, we're having pizza tomorrow." I also recommended: "I hear you're saying you're hungry. This is what you can have." These phrases established Abby's authority and reinforced the family's reliance on the nightly menu without dismissing Ryan's requests.

Two and a half weeks later, Abby and I met for our second session. Abby couldn't wait to share her good report. "Ryan had a great week with eating," she gushed. She went on to share how, despite ongoing growing pains at dinnertime, Ryan seemed to have had a wonderful appetite and it made a difference in the foods he ate at other meals during the day. He had yogurt a few times for breakfast after neglecting it for months. She was also pleased that he tried two new snacks, cheese crackers and almond butter cracker sandwiches, even though they didn't differ much from his typical range of accepted foods.

She saved the best bit of news for last. Not only did Ryan eat an early lunch at behavioral therapy one day, but he also ate a cheese sandwich on a baguette. Abby had packed it for him assuming he wouldn't even open his lunch box. He had only ever eaten a grilled cheese before, and he was even fickle with that. Because we hadn't yet specifically focused on any interventions to expand Ryan's diet, she was optimistic about how things would unfold once we did. I agreed.

Although Abby was still preoccupied with the volume of food that Ryan ate, it was refreshing to hear her discuss his eating positively. I appreciated that she brought up Ryan's appetite. It was something that I had been thinking about, too.

In an early conversation with Abby, I had begun to suspect that Ryan's current eating schedule wasn't working for him. Hunger is governed primarily by one's circadian rhythm, but it's also influenced by what and when we eat. Ryan's hunger and mealtimes weren't aligning, and his appetite wasn't adapting to his schedule. I was concerned that his constant snacking was interfering with his intake at mealtimes. Over the course of a typical day, Ryan was eating three to six snacks of poor nutritional quality and very little at mealtimes. Children who have poor appetites for breakfast, lunch or dinner may be filling up on snacks. As of 2010, American kids were snacking on junk food three times daily, which accounted for more than 27 percent of their daily caloric intake. Furthermore, children are more likely to consume candy, chips and crackers for snacks than they are fruits and vegetables.[60] This means foods of poor nutritional quality are often overshadowing the more healthful foods that are offered at traditional mealtimes.

I talked to Abby to see where we could make adjustments to the timing of Ryan's meals and snacks. The practicality of reducing his snacking frequency turned out to be low. Abby recognized the flaws in Ryan's routine, but she didn't see viable alternatives. Ryan couldn't opt out of the midmorning snack at school, and it wasn't fair to ask him to sit out during snack time while the rest of his classmates ate. Plus, he seemed hungry for that snack. The rest of Ryan's snacks occurred in the car on the way to and from after-school activities and in behavioral therapy, where food was used as an incentive for good behavior. Abby felt that Ryan, a creature of habit, wouldn't be able to handle changes to this routine. Car snacks, she explained, had become a security blanket that Ryan relied on.

I reviewed the potential detriment of these snacks with Abby, but I sensed that she needed more time before she was ready to make a change, so I suggested alternatives. Could she try serving Ryan his uneaten lunch in the car? What if we replaced some of the pretzels with more nutritious options? Could we eliminate the snacks closer to dinner? My intention wasn't to take away Ryan's favorite foods, but to help him feel more inclined to eat more filling foods during mealtimes.

Abby was willing to incorporate new foods and more nutritious options alongside Ryan's usual pretzel snacks, but she wasn't yet ready to trial any further changes. Though I didn't anticipate that her doing so would change Ryan's appetite or nutritional status in a meaningful way, I hoped that encountering new foods would begin to break down his rigidity. I planned to revisit my suggested adjustments later, and in the meantime, we could still work around them to better support Ryan without disrupting his routine.

I next wanted to work with Abby on making adjustments to the location and timing of Ryan's mealtime environment to incorporate more structure and the consistency he thrived on. I felt these modifications would help Ryan specifically, but they're known to be effective in supporting children in general. Kids who grow up with less regulated mealtimes are fussier eaters and tend to enjoy food less than those whose mealtimes have more routine. Additionally, structure is known to help children better attend and respond to hunger cues.[61]

Abby was again attracted to the idea of adding more routine to Ryan's mealtimes, and she agreed that revamping their dinnertime was a much-needed change. As things were, Ryan ate dinner at the kitchen counter or on the couch in the living room. When he ate at the counter, Abby kept him company. Often Ryan's one-year-old sister was eating dinner at the same time as Ryan at the other end of the counter, but because she ate different food and took longer to eat, they didn't really eat together. Ryan's meals were quick, just ten to fifteen minutes, and they were often haphazard, starting with whatever components Abby could prepare quickly and ending with her confirming—a few times—that Ryan didn't want one more bite.

The simplest modification to their current routine would be discontinuing dinners on the couch. I knew that the couch was not physically supporting Ryan in the way that he needed to eat comfortably, and I suspected that sitting there also presented distractions that further impeded his eating. Furthermore, I disliked that he sat there alone, which removed him from the company of his mother and sister. Designating the kitchen as the sole eating area would remove all of those detriments while also giving Ryan a constant that he could come to rely on.

Ryan quickly became comfortable sitting at the counter or kitchen table for dinner, seemingly unfazed by the change in his location. His baby sister delighted in the consistent company at their now communal counter. The only hiccup occurred on the few occasions that she tried to reach over and take some of Ryan's pizza. Luckily, it only happened twice, but both times it derailed Ryan's entire meal.

Abby was a little concerned. She worried that his sister's interest in his meal would deter Ryan from eating altogether. I agreed that he would benefit from as little interference as possible as we sought to modify his diet and mealtime routines, but I still wanted Ryan to continue eating alongside his sister. She had a robust appetite and her enthusiasm for eating could be influential. I encouraged Abby to brush the food-snatching episodes aside and tried to shift the focus. Shared meals were valuable. These altercations were not barriers but learning opportunities for both kids.

Children who participate in regular shared meals are more likely to enjoy healthy weight and eating patterns and are less likely to have disordered eating.[62] Just as importantly, mealtimes impact all of our senses. The sight, touch, taste and smell of food and the shared conversation have positive effects on eating habits and family relationships.[63] Family meals also offer the opportunity to spend time together and communicate with and listen to each other. I could already see that Ryan and his sister were beginning to understand how to negotiate shared space and food. Ryan was learning how to accommodate the disruptions that arose when eating with others, just as his sister was learning to respect boundaries.

Our next session was scheduled for nearly a month after Abby had first introduced the visual menu. At this point, Ryan was no longer requesting pizza for dinner every single night. Abby still served it several times a week and it was still his favorite, but he was more accustomed to expecting his dinner instead of dictating what it was. Although Ryan's frequent snacking was unchanged, he was more regularly accepting grilled cheese, cheese sandwiches and yogurt, which added more nutritious variety to his diet. Overall, Abby was feeling more optimistic.

With Ryan's improved comfort at mealtimes and growing flexibility with his diet, I sat down with Abby to finally address direct strategies for introducing Ryan to new foods. We started with the basics of when and how. Given Ryan's tendency to not eat a lot at one time, it seemed important to offer new foods when he was hungriest. I suggested Abby focus on serving new foods with breakfast, in the moments before dinner when she was preparing his meal, in the car after school and for dinner. Additionally, I reviewed Kay Toomey's progressive steps that lead from simply tolerating foods to finally eating, and I advised her to serve small portions and offer only one new food at a time.

Then, given what I knew about Ryan, I thought that alongside these practical strategies, he would also benefit from the opportunity to get involved with new foods outside of mealtimes. Ryan never hesitated to engage with foods that fell outside of his umbrella of accepted items. Abby told me that he tended to request foods that he saw in his favorite storybook or TV characters enjoying, but he never actually ate them. Similarly, Ryan found it exciting to encounter new foods during the family's twice weekly grocery shopping trips. He held on to new foods that he found appealing, but declined Abby's offers to taste them once he was home.

I identified food shopping, already a part of their routine, as an effective way to increase Ryan's incentive to eat. I hoped that if we could couple his interest in the behind-the-scenes aspects of eating with hands-on food activities, that he would acquire the inclination and comfort to eventually eat new foods. I gave Abby suggestions for activities that would capitalize on Ryan's curiosity and facilitate bringing him from the grocery store to the kitchen, where they could prepare and eventually taste their findings.

The first was a scavenger hunt. I created a list of foods for Ryan to find in the grocery store. Then, to take it a step further, I recommended that Abby and Ryan use the foods they found in the scavenger hunt in an *Iron Chef* challenge at home—they would cook the scavenger hunt food for an upcoming meal.

All of my usual recommendations for engaging with new foods still applied. Ryan was not required to taste or even touch anything that he wasn't yet ready to. I hoped that he would be more open to engaging once he was involved in fun interactions with food than he was when he passively encountered them on his plate. When kids engage with food in the ways I was suggesting that Ryan do, they are more likely to eat and have positive associations with the food. Letting kids use all of their senses to explore food gives them positive experiences and inspires them to taste foods they're initially skeptical of. Researchers believe that one reason creative sensory-based food activities are so effective is because they instill a joy of eating, even among picky eaters.[64]

Abby and I had planned to reconvene just a week later, but her whole family got sick and we ended up delaying until it had been well over twice that long. Although Abby hadn't been able to give the plan the try she had been hoping for due to illness, she reported some small wins. She and Ryan had two good trips to the grocery store. From his scavenger hunt list, Ryan found cherries ("a smooth fruit") and a package of frozen peas ("a frozen vegetable"). At home, Abby put Ryan in charge of washing the cherries, and she began to regularly serve one cherry with Ryan's breakfast so he had the opportunity to try it when he was ready.

The peas had a lot of potential, but after they got home, Ryan was reluctant to take Abby's suggestions to try them both frozen and defrosted. Later that day, Abby checked in with me for ideas on what to try. We discussed mashing the peas with Parmesan cheese to make a green dip, which Ryan could eat with chips. Because he was in a dipping phase and sometimes ate guacamole and hummus, this preparation might feel familiar to him.

Later that week, Abby asked Ryan to help her defrost the peas in the microwave to make the green dip. She served it with chips right in the kitchen as soon as they finished preparing it. She tried it first, telling Ryan about what she thought of the texture and flavor.

Given Ryan's history of avoiding new foods, I had advised Abby that he might benefit from hearing about how new foods tasted before he tried them. I recommended that she create connections between the new food and his preferred ones so he could learn what to expect. "Hmm...it's soft and creamy like hummus and guacamole," she told him, "but it's not completely smooth and has more pieces than hummus." She told him it was also a little cheesy. Abby took another taste and offered Ryan a chip so he could try for himself. He dipped the chip and took a small taste. Although he didn't say anything and wasn't inclined to try another bite, Abby and I agreed this was a big accomplishment for their first attempt.

In the weeks since I had first recommended that she incorporate food shopping and cooking with him, Abby had also managed to find other opportunities to begin nudging Ryan out of his dietary comfort zone. Once he got over being sick, she began including a small portion, between the size of a pea and a penny, of one new food on his plate at mealtimes. Ryan didn't protest the additions, and after a few meals he began to look at and occasionally poke them. His biggest accomplishment occurred the night Abby served him two pieces of tortellini with a small bowl of sauce on the side. "He picked one up, smelled it, licked it and even nibbled on some of the plain dough. That's big!" Abby told me. "I was really proud of him."

Abby and I next met for a check-in three weeks later. At this point, we had been working together for about two months, and she understood the fundamental strategies for optimizing Ryan's meals and intake. I wanted to hear about Ryan's progress before introducing any further tactics. Moving forward would likely just be a matter of tweaking and creating a long-term plan.

Listening to Abby's updates, I noticed that it sounded like Ryan's attitude toward new foods was evolving. His gut reaction was no longer to avoid items he didn't want. He was instead opting to engage with them with increasing frequency. He was regularly picking up, smelling and licking new foods. Additionally, he was continuing to reintegrate formerly preferred foods and was beginning to branch out on variations of his staples.

For example, he had started to eat cream cheese and jelly sandwiches that Abby packed for him to have as a late lunch after school at therapy. One day he asked Abby for dried pineapple and had consistently been eating it since. Since the day Ryan ate the baguette and cheese, he was more regularly having cheese sandwiches. He was only eating a few bites at a time, but he always welcomed them. Then, even though he had historically rejected veggie straws, he ate them one night after a swimming lesson before dinner, and they had since moved securely into accepted food territory. Finally, Ryan had also been requesting junk food and snacks less often. Abby agreed that things were looking up.

Knowing that Ryan was now making definitive progress, I wanted to provide Abby with some ideas to further diversify his diet. Because Ryan was already embracing unique variations of his favorite foods—for example, accepting cheese sandwiches and new breads when he used to only eat melted cheese and regular white bread—we contemplated additional ways to incorporate incentives for him to explore more novel foods. I suggested offering quesadillas, similar to his favorite grilled cheese, and serving fresh pineapple, which he used to like, again.

Although his newly welcomed veggie straws had no connection to real vegetables beyond the name, Abby and I both saw the potential for them to pave the way to raw carrots, celery or string beans. We created a food chain progressing from the airy veggie sticks to similarly salty puffed pea crisps. From there, we might try freeze-dried string beans and proceed eventually to crunchy fresh string beans, sugar snap peas, carrot sticks, celery and jicama. (Jicama is one of my secret weapons. Though not the most common, it's an easy entry into the vegetable world for picky eaters. Kids enjoy its crunchy, juicy, consistent texture and mildly sweet taste.) The idea was to build on and expand the appearances and textures that Ryan was comfortable with. The similarities to familiar foods would serve as his anchor, allowing him to engage with new foods more comfortably.

Grounded in the idea that there is a reason we eat the foods we do, these strategies were thoughtful supplements to the feeding foundation that Abby already had in place. While they're effective, they take time. I wasn't anticipating an immediate enthusiastic email from Abby reporting that serving similar foods was transformative. As expected, I didn't get one. Ryan didn't methodically progress through the veggie straw food chain we had discussed, but he did warm up to having vegetables on his plate. I reminded Abby that any time Ryan tolerated, touched or otherwise engaged with a novel food, he was taking a meaningful step toward eating a more diverse diet.

Before I started working with Abby and Ryan, Ryan had become selective about the specific brands and presentations of foods that he ate. For example, despite his love for pizza, he only ate one kind, which was why Abby stockpiled slices from his favorite restaurant. In our next session, Abby brought up the preference that she found more difficult to accommodate: Ryan's insistence on eating one particular flavor of yogurt from one brand in one particular package. She was glad that he was eating yogurt again at all, but she found his rigidity limiting. She was hoping to expand his comfort with new brands and flavors and worried that Ryan would be stuck eating the same sugary yogurt from the same tube forever. I assured her this wouldn't be the case.

I suggested she disguise the packaging of his preferred yogurt or try serving it in a different container to break Ryan's brand loyalty and get him accustomed to variety. Then, to address the flavor factor, I recommended mixing an almost undetectable portion of plain with his preferred flavor. The idea was that as Ryan grew comfortable with the combination, Abby could continue to adjust the ratio. Down the line Ryan might accept plain yogurt with fruit or jam or even on its own. This method was also an effective way to introduce him to new yogurt flavors or variations of other foods.

After our discussion, Abby served Ryan yogurt in a small bowl. He didn't eat it. The next time, she offered a new brand in a similar package. Again, he declined. Two months before, Abby would have accepted Ryan's double rejection as just another confirmation that he was picky and would have abandoned future attempts. But with my reminders about the need for repeated exposures echoing in her head, she decided to give it another shot. I've become used to hearing phrases like, "No, she won't do that," "He won't like that," and, "She tried it and didn't like it," when I propose a new food or strategy for a parent to try with a child. These assertions originate from a place of experience. It's true, the child hasn't done that *before*, and they *typically* don't like that. But these incidents aren't set in stone. I tell parents who respond this way what I told Abby numerous times: We need to give children time before taking away their learning opportunities.

Later that week, Ryan ate the new yogurt the second time she offered it. "I realized it was because he wasn't hungry the first time I offered it," Abby shared. She was both humbled and enthused. She had since bought a variety of brands of blueberry yogurt, Ryan's preferred flavor, and he continued to accept them. "It was a good lesson for me," she said. She finally saw how Ryan was more likely to try new foods when he was hungry, and more important, that he wouldn't have the opportunity to do so if she stopped offering them.

Abby's yogurt experience was such a valuable reminder that we can't make rash assumptions about kids' eating. Taking one rejection as truth and failing to provide repeat exposures can deprive children of the opportunity to grow and surprise us. Ultimately, we can't make up our minds about what kids do and don't like.

Abby was actually growing more curious about Ryan's preferences. Yet even as Abby continued to provided Ryan with multiple exposures, she also wondered whether there was a point when she should accept that he simply didn't like something. Essentially, Abby was asking how she could distinguish his neophobia from a true preference. When would it be fair to stop offering a new food?

These were thoughtful questions and important ones to ask, but I didn't have concrete answers for her. I think it's helpful to look at the bigger picture: What is the child's attitude about that food and new foods in general? Is their denial an isolated incident or a pattern in their eating? Did they even try the new food?

I don't advocate for overriding a child's inherent preferences, and I don't believe it's my or a parent's job to manipulate a child's taste buds. In fact, I believe that it is crucial to respect a child's likes and dislikes. But I also believe it is just as necessary to provide kids with ample opportunity to discover what those are and to explore how adaptable they might be.

Abby had actually come to the same conclusion on her own. She was still testing where it made sense to push Ryan, and she was still exploring what both of their limits were. "I'm noticing his preferences coming through and I'm trying to respect them," she told me. For example, a few weeks after Ryan had been accepting cheese sandwiches, he started asking to have the bread toasted. At first Abby resisted his request. Toasted bread wasn't on the menu. But when Ryan's requests persisted, she considered what he was actually asking. His demand wasn't outrageous or unfeasible. He wasn't seeking a completely different meal. In fact, he was trying to work with her to eat the one she served. He was simply saying, "I prefer this a different way. Can we make it happen?" She thought about it and decided they could.

Abby was learning to accommodate those types of compromises. "There are so few things that Ryan can control. He's told what to do for everything," she told me. "His instinct is to challenge what you say, and then when you agree with him, he's shocked." So, she was discovering more ways that she could be lenient within their framework and it was paying off. For example, one evening Ryan protested the peanut butter sandwich Abby was about to serve, requesting instead a plain piece of bread and peanut butter on a spoon. "It's basically a sandwich," Abby decided when she told me about the incident. "Why should I care if he preferred them separately?" It didn't change the nutritional essence of what he was eating, it didn't upset their division of responsibility and it wasn't an outrageous request. So, she let him have bread and peanut butter instead of the sandwich. She didn't think it mattered and wanted to know if I agreed. I did.

I appreciated Abby's perspective. Our intention was never to teach Ryan to eat everything, but for him to be flexible with food, to eat enough and to enjoy a nutritious variety. Whether he was eating the peanut butter in a sandwich or on a spoon, Ryan was becoming less rigid. With the right balance of limits and lenience, I was confident that his diet would continue to grow. Ultimately, mealtimes had become a dance between the two of them—Abby urging Ryan to broaden his boundaries, using his responses to inform her next move, and Ryan asserting his preferences and acquiring new ones. Together, they were finding a rhythm that worked for them both.

When we had first met, Abby told me that Ryan had become "insanely picky" over the past year. With Ryan now showing signs of progress, Abby began to wonder whether he actually wasn't as selective as she thought. Maybe it's a personality thing, she wondered. "He's never been a food person. He's just not someone who's that interested in eating."

She questioned whether Ryan's appetite was the true barrier. Maybe, she suggested, Ryan is just a kid who doesn't have a hearty appetite and doesn't love to eat. Abby wasn't wrong to consider the potential implications of Ryan's appetite. I agreed that it could be a factor in his food choices. But I hoped that Abby was realizing that she didn't need to coerce Ryan into eating something he didn't want to. It wasn't her responsibility, just as his intake wasn't a marker of his progress. If Ryan did experience variability in his hunger and had periods when he required less food, he seemed to be honoring the messages that his body was sending him.

When I met Ryan, he lacked the flexibility that he needed to eat comfortably and subsequently had atypical intake and a limited food repertoire. I didn't think these impairments were simply a manifestation of low appetite. Eating difficulties are usually multifactorial. Moreover, if Abby began to focus too much on the potential ramifications of Ryan's appetite, it could distract her from the efforts that were helping and would continue to help him.

I believe that every child deserves the opportunity to enjoy food and to eat without restrictions or reservations, and I believed that Ryan needed ongoing support to get to that point. He was making real progress. He was welcoming new foods and becoming more flexible with his menu. I think that was why Abby started looking to his appetite. Ryan was no longer the "insanely picky" kid that she once knew. His progress wasn't a sign that he didn't need help. Instead, it was evidence that the approaches were working and that his eating habits would continue to improve.

Activity: Grocery Games

Including a child in tangential eating activities is an engaging way to help them gain more exposure to new foods and spark their appreciation for and interest in these foods. This is an exciting supplemental activity to the basic foundation of and efforts that occur during mealtimes. It is a chance for kids to have a positive experience with food. When they're in the store instead of at the table, they might touch or consider things they normally would not.

Try these grocery store games to pique your child's interest and help them develop a positive relationship with food. Adapt as necessary to suit your child's age and interests.

Mystery Foods: Collect a few items in the basket at the grocery store without letting your child see what they are. Have your child shut their eyes as they explore the foods in their hands and try to identify each item based on its size, weight, shape and smell.

Grocery Scavenger Hunt: Turn grocery shopping into a scavenger hunt. You can use this activity to complete your regular grocery list or make it a game by using some of the ideas below or thinking of your own. Find:

- A food that starts with the first letter of your name
- A vegetable that comes in two different colors
- A food listed as "organic"
- A frozen vegetable
- Three foods that start with the letter "___"
- A food that you can't eat raw

- The ingredients to make meatballs/lasagna/chicken soup/etc.
- One fruit or vegetable from every color of the rainbow
- A fruit that is smooth
- A fruit that is bumpy
- A protein you've never tried before
- A condiment you've never seen before
- Two different kinds of chicken
- Something you can't pronounce
- One fruit and one vegetable that are purple
- A vegetable with a peel
- Three items made from grains
- Cheese shaped like a circle
- Cheese shaped like a square
- A food you've never tried before
- A food you love to eat
- A food you'd like to try
- A food that doesn't need to be cooked
- A food with a nice smell
- Something that your parent/caregiver likes to eat
- A vegetable in a can
- A pasta shape you've never seen before
- Ingredients to make a sandwich
- Three different flavors of yogurt

Color Finder: Provide your child with a color and then have them identify all of the items they can find in that color. Provide each child with a different color and keep score if you're shopping with a sibling or friend. As a bonus, pick one to take home to sample or incorporate into a recipe that you select together. If your child is not ready to eat yet, go online or to the library to learn more about the food. Some kids might also like to create a story or make an art project incorporating the food.

Iron Chef: At the grocery store, your child can select one or two foods that must be included in the next meal. You can get very creative and try to include one item in every dish.

Breaking Boundaries: At the supermarket, ask your child to pick out a fruit or vegetable they have never seen before or have never eaten at home. Take this new food home. Select a recipe to prepare together.

Would You Rather: While you're shopping, select a few pairs of ingredients and ask your child which they would rather eat. An apple or a pear? Yogurt or cottage cheese? Pesto or tomato sauce? Try this with new and preferred foods. You might find one they're willing to take home.

Guess the Dish: Gather all of the ingredients needed to make a familiar meal. Can your child guess what you're making? Try this the other way around, too. Have your child guess all of the ingredients required to make a meal you have planned.

CHAPTER 6

Double Trouble
Picky Eater Siblings

Heather had three main challenges when it came to mealtimes with her kids. First, meals were stressful. With her concerns about whether and how much her children ate, she confessed that meals were her least favorite part of her day. Second, she didn't like to cook, and she struggled with what to make. Both of her children were particular, both had unique dietary restrictions and both were bored with their limited diets, even though they were resistant to trying new foods. Finally, meals seemed to last an eternity, and evenings felt too short. By the time everyone arrived home from after-school activities, they only had three hours to cook, eat, bathe and get to bed.

Ultimately, Heather told me, the family was struggling to make room for the long forty-five minutes during which she and her husband held their breath hoping the kids ate without a fuss. Rarely was that the case. More often, their young daughter was whining at the table and their son would leave his plate to rummage through the kitchen looking for what he deemed a suitable alternative to the meal on the table.

Heather also had concerns about the kids' diet quality. In the months before calling me, Heather had turned her focus to optimizing what her kids ate. Looking at their predominantly processed diets, she began to wonder whether poor nutrition could be exacerbating behaviors they struggled with. Both Chloe, who was approaching five when we started working together, and Peter, eighteen months older, had special needs. Heather struggled to manage them and she knew they struggled every day, too.

Chloe and Peter's diets weren't atrocious when you looked at the numbers. Each ate more than fifteen substantial foods, many of which were fruit, plus several snacks and sweets. However, their diets lacked diversity, and between the two of them, there were few meaningful overlaps. The disparity fueled Heather's distress. Frozen chicken nuggets, macaroni and cheese and pizza were the only three meals that both kids would eat for lunch or dinner, though Peter frequently protested the dairy-free versions that Chloe ate due to sensitivities.

For breakfast, their overlap extended only to a particular brand of French toast sticks and waffles. Both liked SunButter, blackberries, strawberries, blueberries and apples, and both only ate vegetables if they were pureed and came in a pouch. Of course, to Heather's frustration, they preferred different flavors. The rest of their intake was filled almost exclusively with packaged frozen products, like French fries (both) and fish sticks (Chloe). Other than a protein shake with frozen fruit that Chloe ate, nothing was fresh or close to homemade.

Chloe had eaten well as a toddler, but for the past three years her interest in food had waned. She ate very little throughout the day and had trouble sitting still during meals, though based on her growth trends, her intake appeared sufficient. She couldn't tolerate nonpre-ferred foods on her plate, and lately, despite never before having any difficulty manipulating a texturally diverse diet, she had begun to gravitate to softer foods, abandoning former favorites like rice cakes. On top of that, she was doing peculiar things like nibbling the breading off of chicken nuggets, chewing with her front teeth and spitting out partially chewed bits of food. Based on previous evaluations, Chloe was identified as a sensory avoider, someone who overreacted to sensory input. Lately it seemed like her sensitivities had intensified.

Similar to his sister, Peter became picky around the age of two. For most of his life now, he had restricted his diet to a small selection of foods, which was further limited by his allergies to eggs, sesame, peanuts and tree nuts. Unlike Chloe, he was a sensory seeker, had a great appetite and seemed to always be hungry, though only for his specific collection of preferred foods.

Peter didn't really eat protein. It was a milestone when he started eating chicken nuggets a year ago and pizza a few months prior to Heather's reaching out to me. Much to her frustration, Peter rejected foods based solely on sight and smell. In addition to the probable sensory factor, there was a behavioral component to his resistance. Heather believed Peter was more capable of eating than his limited diet suggested. In fact, since recently beginning feeding therapy with an occupational therapist, Peter had eaten two new foods, a few bites of a hot dog and grilled chicken strips. Peter wasn't interested when Heather incorporated them into his meals at home, so these accomplishments had yet to contribute to meaningful change in his daily diet.

Like any mom, Heather wanted her kids to thrive. Curious if there might be room for improvement if they ate more nutritious foods and fewer processed ones, Heather had both kids tested for food sensitivities. The findings uncovered a number of potential offenders for each, and while the results seemed promising, they ultimately didn't ease things as she had hoped. Attempting to adhere to the myriad of suggested restrictions left her kids with little to eat.

When she temporarily eliminated some of their essentials, their intake plummeted. To make things worse, because their suspected sensitivities had little overlap, everything from grocery shopping to cooking became even more difficult and time-consuming. Though they were limited,

Heather missed the kids' preferred foods just as much as the kids did, and she wasn't even sure they felt or behaved any better after having been without them for a few days.

At this time, she realized that in order to optimize Chloe and Peter's health, she needed to address the underlying issues that were interfering with their ability to eat outside of their comfort zones. Her short-lived attempts to change their diets highlighted how arduous it was to feed her kids, not just more nutritious foods but anything. That's when she reached out to me.

Based on my preliminary conversations with Heather, I saw opportunity for improvement in mealtime logistics and how the family interacted during meals. All three of Heather's concerns were valid. Mealtimes weren't working. She wanted mealtimes to be quicker and to feel more relaxed. She wanted to make one menu for the whole family. Yet as things were, meals were not supporting Heather's priorities, and they did not look or feel as she had envisioned. They were too long, too lax and too stressful. Ultimately, though her kids were eating, they weren't eating well. No one was truly content, and no one felt like meals were a success.

Heather had two goals: to make mealtimes less stressful and to expand the range of foods that her children ate. I agreed that broadening Chloe and Peter's diets would likely eliminate much of the stress Heather experienced at mealtimes, but I sensed that the stress derived from the fact that the structure and tone of the kids' meals was not productive. I didn't want to neglect opportunities for improvement in their current routine by focusing strictly on the food, so I recommended we focus on mealtimes first.

As Heather and I dove into more details about the family's mealtimes in our first full session, I learned that the kids ate together, having breakfast at the counter and eating dinner at the table, where Chloe was able to sit for longer before fussing or losing interest. Heather and her husband ate breakfast on the go and joined the kids for dinner if there was time after they had prepared their own meal. The kids each had a separate meal, and Heather often accommodated their special requests mid-meal so that they could end their days feeling full and satisfied. Although Heather wished the kids ate differently, she never cajoled or bargained with them to make this happen. Still, she was known to suggest one more bite and encourage the kids to eat more of the nutritious foods they tended to avoid.

I believe that positive, pressure-free meals are at the foundation of raising children who like to eat and have a rewarding relationship with food—even for those at the extreme end of the picky eating spectrum. I also believe that positivity and lack of pressure don't mean a lack of structure or routine. Clarity and boundaries regarding the logistics of mealtimes are crucial for enabling kids to thrive at the table. Research shows that children's eating suffers when there is either *too much* or *not enough* attention on what and how they eat. When parents delegate too many decisions to their children or fail to accommodate their children's needs and preferences, children eat poorly. In the same vein, children don't eat well when parents micromanage.[65] The key is finding the sweet spot between rigidity and lenience.

Structured mealtimes with clear expectations and an appropriate amount of freedom provide children with the optimal environment for both eating and learning. I understand that the natural response to seeing a child struggle with food and repeatedly refuse to eat is to do anything necessary to help them eat more comfortably. Heather had done this, as any parent would, but she had done so at the expense of permitting her kids to dominate mealtimes in a way that ultimately wasn't providing the results that she hoped for.

Ellyn Satter, creator of the Division of Responsibility for Feeding, writes in her book *Child of Mine* that when it comes to feeding, "it is important to matter-of-factly set the limits and avoid the emotional fireworks and struggles."[66] Food limits were few in Heather's household. The kids largely determined their diets and set the tone for mealtimes. If Heather failed to incorporate more structure into her feeding approach, her desire to make mealtimes more pleasant and to expand the range of foods that her kids ate were unlikely to come to fruition.

I had two initial suggestions to help Heather reach her goals. I wanted to redefine each family member's role regarding eating and feeding, and I wanted to create opportunities for her children to meet and engage with novel foods. We started that day with mealtime roles.

I explained to Heather that if she and her husband clearly defined what they and the kids were accountable for when it came to what, when and how they ate, then meals would feel less hectic and would flow more efficiently. This sort of structure would also create opportunities for diet expansion, which I planned to address in a future session.

Although it would be an adjustment for the kids, Peter in particular, I recommended that Heather and her husband oversee the what, where and when of feeding. That meant that they would select the menu, mealtime location and daily meal schedule. Once the food was on the table, Chloe and Peter could then decide how much they wanted to eat and whether they even wanted to eat at all.

This framework, based on Satter's Division of Responsibility for Feeding, supposes that kids are able to attend to their own hunger when they are supported with regularly scheduled meals and appropriate foods. However, parents of children with eating difficulties know that kids don't always "eventually eat." Some kids have difficulty regulating their intake. Others are more comfortable not eating than eating something or somewhere that just isn't right.

Even for children with aversions this extreme, I still advocate that families follow this model or some iteration of it. The presence of extreme eating difficulties does not necessitate complete permissiveness on the parents' part. Instead, each child's unique presentation can invite special accommodations within the basic framework, a compromise that gives a child support in all of the areas they need to eat adequately and comfortably, while still creating structure in their routine and space for improvement in their eating.

Heather, practical and level-headed, embraced the theory behind my recommendations without hesitation or question. While she acknowledged the potential stress they might inspire in her children, Heather believed the adjustments would eventually work for her family. She expected Peter to resist the limitations on his fridge foraging, but she didn't anticipate a hunger strike. She was more concerned about the impact on Chloe's intake. We agreed to keep an eye on it, which left Heather feeling confident introducing the new routine. She believed that when she did, her children would eventually welcome it as well.

At the end of our first session, we discussed Heather's plan to transition to the new mealtime protocol. When she shared the adjustments with the kids, I didn't want Chloe or Peter to feel that they were being punished or that their autonomy was being taken away. Highlighting their ongoing agency in what and how much they ate was crucial for helping them feel safe with the new routine and especially as they began to encounter and eventually explore novel foods. Just as the kids needed to respect the boundaries that their parents set, Heather and her husband were to accept and respect their children's appetites and preferences, which meant that as hard as it may be, Heather needed to avoid expressing her concern over how much her kids ate.

I told Heather that the stressful days of pleading with Chloe and Peter, urging them to take a bite and asking if they were completely sure that they had had enough were done. The new roles were in place to ensure no one would feel a sense of pressure related to food. The kids were never going to have to eat something they were uncomfortable with, and they would never be expected to eat more or less than what felt right at any one time. Even if it was coming from a good place—of wanting to ensure that her kids were full and satisfied—Heather's focus on what and how much they ate could further deter Chloe and Peter from eating, and that's exactly what she was seeking to avoid.

As much as the divisions and expectations made sense to her, Heather admitted that the largest adjustment might be her own. Letting go during mealtimes and releasing her intrinsic concern about the quality of her kids' dinner intake were counter to everything she had known for the past four years. I appreciated her perspective and honesty. While I agreed that there would probably be growing pains for everyone, I assured her that once the adjustment period passed, she would be released from the burden of hoping that her kids ate and would finally feel better about what they did consume. Once the structure was in place and everyone was comfortable in their roles, meals would flow naturally and enjoyably, and from there, she could experience more pleasant mealtimes and could finally see improvement in the quality and variety of her kids' diets.

When Heather and I met two weeks later, she shared that Chloe and Peter were receptive to the idea of the new plan. They enjoyed hearing that they were in control of what they ate from the table, but when they actually sat down to a meal, they found following the new guidelines to be challenging.

Peter required reinforcement with the "what" of mealtimes. Because he had been accustomed to heading into the kitchen mid-meal to select his own foods, losing this freedom felt restrictive. He tested his limits. He tried several times over the course of the week to leave the table in search of alternatives, but Heather, a no-nonsense mom, didn't give in. The family was trying something new and sticking with it, she told them.

When she pointed out to Peter that nothing fundamental had changed about his meals, that she was not requiring him to do anything different, that he still had access to his favorite foods and that he didn't have to eat anything he wasn't ready to, he eventually acquiesced. The task of remaining at the table wasn't challenging for him in and of itself. It was easier than feeding therapy, where he was persuaded to sample novel foods. It was the idea that didn't sit well with him. Although he would have preferred to have free rein in the kitchen, and though he continued to periodically test his boundaries, he ultimately adjusted to the new routine.

Chloe continued to struggle to maintain her attention and stay still in her seat throughout the duration of the meal. I didn't see an immediate resolution to her fidgeting. She already had an ideal chair that provided support at her hips, knees and feet. The family already ate without tempting distractions like the TV. I also didn't blame her for the impulse to move around. Protracted meals had become the family's norm, not because the kids were remarkably slow eaters but because they spent so much time unfocused, fussy and not actively eating. Heather and her husband also contributed when they checked in to see that the kids were eating enough and urged them to consider an additional bite or two. Ultimately, the forty-five minutes that their meals took was too long of a time to expect Chloe to sit comfortably. Young kids need no more than twenty to thirty minutes at the table for full meals, but even that, I imagined, would be a stretch for Chloe.

Reasoning with a five-year-old (*it's a whole twenty minutes less that you're used to, you can do that*) was an unreasonable approach to improving Chloe's tableside endurance. Instead, I suggested that Heather give Chloe incremental tasks that she could easily accomplish, adjust to and then continue to build on. I advised Heather to invest in a visual timer that clearly illustrated passing and remaining time. At first, she could set the timer for five minutes, during which Chloe had to sit. Then, Chloe could take a short break if she needed. After the break, Chloe was to return to the table to eat for another five minutes and then repeat the whole cycle until the meal was finished.

Gradually, as Chloe adjusted to five minutes of focused eating time, Heather could increase the seating time—five minutes could become seven, then ten, etc.—and, as Chloe continued to gain her table endurance, she would also incrementally decrease the break time until she was ultimately able to sit for the entire duration of a meal, twenty to thirty minutes. "I'm ready for this," Heather said when I suggested the timer. She had been craving shorter and more cohesive meals and couldn't hide her delight in the additional fifteen to twenty-five minutes they would gain in the evenings once they condensed mealtimes.

Having addressed the structural logistics about how to manage mealtimes, Heather and I moved on to the next components of her mealtime makeover: eating as a family and introducing new foods. Because Chloe and Peter were already eating together and because they were comfortable being around nonpreferred foods, I figured we could bundle these steps together.

Sharing family meals was one of Heather's specific goals, but it's also a ritual I encourage every family I work with to adopt because of the impact eating together can have in shaping a child's development and eating habits. Beyond contributing to improved nutritional intake, family meals create the opportunity for children to absorb vital social skills—how to share, how to participate in and make conversation, how to pass and serve food, how to say no thank you and yes please and how to express their pleasures and dislikes in a constructive and unoffending way.[67,68] Luckily, improved eating is a common side effect of fulfilling interactions with family; children eat well when all of their needs are met.

Making a single meal for a family that includes picky eaters with unique dietary restrictions doesn't imply disregarding individual needs and preferences. Caregivers have a duty to create an eating environment that is safe and appropriate for their children. This means accommodating the family's dietary needs while also considering their preferences. A meal does not feel safe to a picky eater if it lacks a safe food. Therefore, the key to transitioning from preparing distinct meals to a shared one is including a substantial portion of at least one food that each diner will always eat at every meal, even if they will be the only one eating it. A shared meal can include any number of an individual's preferred foods, but, as I told Heather, a minimum of one is all that is needed.

I don't suggest this potentially drastic and triggering mealtime transformation without compassion for the reasons behind how separate menus for picky eaters came to be. Children with eating difficulties have legitimate reasons for eating and resisting the foods they do.

Heather and I agreed that, despite their aversions and unique needs, her kids would likely transition to sharing family-style meals without major hiccups. Chloe was averse to having nonpreferred foods on her plate, but she didn't mind having them around her. Peter resisted eating new foods, but similarly did not have difficulty tolerating their proximity. Furthermore, they were used to eating together, sometimes even with their parents, and each sibling did not always eat foods that the other liked. Therefore, Heather and I anticipated that Chloe and Peter could both comfortably transition to eating alongside nonpreferred foods in their new dinner routine.

Next, we discussed the details of serving a single menu. Peter and Chloe had enough overlapping foods—a few mains and a selection of fruits and sides like applesauce, French fries and white bread—that the transition to making one shared meal for the family instead of three separate ones wouldn't be overly complicated for Heather. In fact, little beyond the presentation and timing had to change. She and her husband could continue eating their usual meals—usually prepared selections from a delivery service—but rather than prepare the kids' dinners first and join them later on, I recommended the family sit down together at the same time. And instead of pre-plating, I recommended serving from communal dishes to further erode the dis-tinctions of "Chloe's food" or "Mom and Dad's food." My intention was that every food on the table would be an "everyone" dish. Everyone might not be ready to eat it yet, but I wanted to send the message that eventually they would be.

The only complication was that their parents' food didn't regularly accommodate Chloe and Peter's food restrictions. Additionally, because their parents routinely ate a varied menu of prepared meals, family meals would not provide the repeated exposure that Chloe and Peter needed to develop new preferences. So, I talked to Heather about setting them up for success by serving one specific new food per meal that we would select specifically to help Chloe and Peter expand their diets. In other words, I wanted Heather to serve a goal food that they would be most likely to eat.

I envisioned something that would equally benefit and appeal to both Chloe and Peter. Chloe gravitated to soft, easy-to-chew, bland foods that didn't have diverse texture. Like so many kids' diets, hers lacked diversity, though to my surprise she was currently eating at least one food from every food group. Peter, on the other hand, welcomed more textural diversity, but had yet to find a protein that he regularly enjoyed.

I anticipated both kids would appreciate the starchiness, mild flavor and textural simplicity of beans, and I anticipated that Heather would appreciate that they did not require complex preparation. The simple act of opening a can wouldn't tax their already busy evenings. To avoid monotony, I recommended that Heather introduce three types of beans over the course of a week. Similarly, I suggested that she rotate the kids' daily menus to avoid serving the same foods two days in a row. The more variety Chloe and Peter encountered, the more open they would be to incorporating new foods into their repertoires. Inspired by the kids' preferences for ketchup, carbs and sweets, we opted to rotate red kidney beans and baked beans, hoping that these would make for an easy entry to a world of new food.

I told Heather that the kids could have as much of their preferred food—or any food on the table—as they wanted. Whatever and however much they chose to eat was their decision and theirs only. Though there would never be an obligation for the kids to try new foods, I didn't want them to ignore the variety of foods they would be encountering on the table. Instead, I wanted to encourage interactions that would facilitate their learning, and more importantly, I wanted to teach them that eating could be fun.

I recommended that moving forward, everyone would serve themselves a portion of every food on the table. Neither the kids nor the parents would be obligated to eat the food or even put it anywhere near their mouths. If they didn't want it on their plates, they could place it on their place mat or a napkin close by. However, the kids had a new responsibility to initiate a fun interaction with the goal food. Yes, I told Heather, they not only could, but should, play with their food.

Many extreme picky eaters have a deeply negative relationship with nonpreferred foods. One of my primary goals in working with them is to replace negative experiences with gratifying ones. The picky eater's path to a future of positive food experiences is unlikely to be swift or smooth. Whichever way it unfolds, however long it takes, I believe it's paved with pleasurable, pressure-free interactions with food. To this end, I've suggested activities as prosaic as reading books about food, playing with food models, surveying recipes and grocery shopping. Anything that reveals the joy of food and eating is welcome.

Yet, my preferred solution for achieving these fun, low-pressure interactions—playing with food—is a bit more involved. Food play harnesses kids' inherent inclination to have fun. When a child is playing, they can engage in a way that they might not otherwise. These fun interactions build familiarity and comfort with new foods that can eventually bridge the gap to eating. Think of a child who may refuse to look at a novel food. When they understand that there is no expectation that they eat, and the food transforms from a threat to a character in their pretend play land, they can suddenly embrace the opportunity to engage in a much more intimate way than they otherwise would have.

This is what makes food play so effective. When a child is truly immersed in play, they are no longer in an eating mindset. When they are instead involved in an experience that is filled with pleasure and wonder, the door to eating actually opens. Food becomes less scary and more approachable. That is precisely our goal.

The idea of playing with food tends to rub people the wrong way. We're taught to be neat and polite when eating, so it's counter to how we culturally address food. Having food on your face is viewed as a major faux pas during a meal, but it's one of my favorite ways to play. I don't suggest manners go out the window, but when encouraging extreme picky eaters to break down their food objections, I believe it is valuable to be lenient on the tidiness front and embrace both the mess and the joy that accompany creative exploration.

That being said, it is reasonable to encourage kids to explore food in ways that are appropriate for the table. I leave what that looks like up to the individual household, but I do encourage families to embrace the mess. At the very least, I recommend they check their urge to clean and keep things tidy. Hindering a picky eater's play in the name of teaching them manners or limiting the cleanup burden will impede their progress. Even worse, frequently wiping food mess from a child's body can actually condition them to dislike being messy and can exacerbate sensory defensiveness. Although I don't believe that the level of mess that one can create or tolerate is directly related to the quality of their relationship with food, I encourage kids and parents to be as messy as they can tolerate.

No matter how fun we perceive hands-on experiences with food to be and no matter how beneficial we know they are, we shouldn't expect hesitant eaters to dive headfirst into carefree play. As they do with eating, picky kids and those with sensory impairments will have the same barriers to overcome before willingly engaging with unfamiliar foods. Therefore, the keys to successful play are to keep the pressure off, avoid forcing an interaction that is above the child's current stage of engagement and keep it fun. I recommend allowing kids to dictate the pace and intensity of their involvement. My rule of thumb, wherever the child is at and whatever their barrier for entry, is for parents to serve as the play guides by initiating and modeling interactions themselves. Following their parents' lead, kids can then observe, imitate and begin to forge their own exploration. From there, the art of parent-led play is to elevate a child's interaction to progressively involve more sensory engagement and move the food closer to the face and mouth. The ultimate goal is to encourage play that allows for smelling, licking and tasting—all big steps for a picky eater and all ones that ultimately lead to eating.

To initiate play with Chloe and Peter, I advised Heather to first demonstrate the activity and encourage their imitation. Be creative and get silly, I told her. Bring in a sense of whimsy. Incorporate their interests. Rather than implore them to engage with a new food, propose an irresistible invitation to have fun: "Let's see if we can . . . go bowling with meatballs, build a log cabin with string beans, paint our nails with pesto, play the asparagus flute."

Heather and I felt that as long as there were no suggestions of eating, Chloe and Peter would warm up to food play, but I still provided Heather with troubleshooting techniques just in case. If the kids were hesitant to make direct contact, they could use a napkin or utensil as a buffer between themselves and their food. If any level of contact was out of the question, or if time or patience were running short, they could instead opt to talk about the food's objective sensory properties by describing the color, shape or size. This would still help break down the kids' negative preconceptions while giving them a more productive way to think about food.

Finally, I recommended that Heather try to find room for additional opportunities to engage with food. But, given how tight she felt weekdays were, I proposed that at a minimum she set aside a few minutes during meals to play with goal foods.

Heather started implementing shared family meals with new foods immediately after we first discussed them. We were in touch frequently over this time. She told me in an email just a few days in that Chloe and Peter easily adjusted to and actually enjoyed sitting as a family. After all, it wasn't a completely new routine for them. Engaging with new foods was a little different.

When Heather told the kids that each night at dinner they'd be passing around a bowl of beans and that everyone would need to serve themselves a portion, Peter responded nonchalantly. Though Heather could see that Chloe had reservations, she waited for her brother's response and ultimately took the announcement in stride as well.

However, when Heather also shared that they should play with the beans on their plate, the kids were less enthusiastic. They didn't initiate play. So, attempting to serve as models, Heather and her husband each squished a bean between their fingers. When Chloe and Peter didn't respond, Heather took a few more and mashed them with her fork.

During our call, Heather told me that Chloe wanted nothing to do with the beans. But as she described Chloe's behavior, I saw that wasn't actually true. The first night, when Chloe resisted squishing the bean, she instead picked one up with her fingers and put it on the tablecloth beside her. Then, Heather told me that the next night, still not yet ready to play, Chloe buried a bean under her macaroni and cheese. Following her lead, Heather did the same and then took it a step further, eating a bean-macaroni combo bite. Chloe watched but continued to eat her own macaroni, careful to leave the portion that was concealing the bean.

Heather relayed that a few days passed with similar interactions. Chloe was engaging but keeping her distance. Chloe had never before touched a bean, and it had been ages since she had eaten or even interacted with a non-preferred food. I saw her first engagement with beans as a productive step in the right direction. Given that she was okay touching and being near the bean, I believed her eating them wasn't too far off.

As for Peter, he also was not open to the idea of playing with beans. Instead, he found a suitable alternative: he ate them. Heather told me that at first he was having just one per night, fulfilling what he deemed to be his minimum requirement. But then, a few nights in, the first night she served baked beans, Peter decided he didn't want the rest of the meal that Heather provided. Unable to forage for alternatives in the kitchen, he ate five baked beans. Heather applauded his accomplishment and proudly reported back to me.

I hoped that Peter's receptivity would play a role in Chloe's and that the kids' individual achievements would inspire the other. Still, I reminded Heather that she needed to be patient. I strongly believed that she would see the improvements that she was looking for, but it would take time, patience and consistency. She couldn't expect them after one dinner, one successful week of food play or even possibly one month. We would continue to tweak the plan as needed, but for now, we needed to give this time.

During the week, Peter got lunch from his school cafeteria. Options were limited due to his food allergies and preferences, but Heather had worked with the school chef to create a menu of new and preferred foods that accommodated Peter's needs.

When Heather and I started our sessions, Peter had been tolerating new foods on his lunch plate daily but was largely ignoring them. However, a few months into the year, when both feeding therapy and the mealtime adjustment that I had recommended were underway, Peter began to make marked progress.

Over the course of a two-week span, he tried salami, whole wheat bread, a beef slider and carrots at school. When Heather told me about his progress, I recommended that she incorporate these newly approved foods into their home menu to build up the exposures he needed to secure his regular consumption.

Around the same time, Peter came home one day reporting that he ate and "really liked" edamame. Heather went out to buy them immediately. Peter ate them happily, and to her total pleasure and surprise, even Chloe put some to her mouth.

Although the kids were at different stages with their eating when they started working with me—Peter was used to interacting with new foods from his time in therapy, and Chloe was averse to having new foods alongside preferred ones on her plate—it seemed their shared participation was serving as a positive influence and support in their upcoming encounters with new foods.

Raising two picky eaters has its pros and cons. On one hand, because siblings have so much sway over each other, picky behavior has the potential to rub off on a more accepting sibling. However, it's just as likely that the more food-tolerant sibling unwittingly sways the pickier eater to embrace more foods. I didn't believe that Chloe's eating struggles had caused Peter's or vice versa. They both had legitimate barriers that led them to engage with food the way they did. I did, however, believe that there was a benefit to their being on the journey of learning to like new foods together.

After a little over a month, the kids' interactions with new foods were picking up. Peter was consistently munching on novel foods. Chloe was playing with them and inviting them into her personal space. Every so often she surprised everyone by taking a bite or licking something new.

Although Chloe and Peter were doing so well with their nightly interactions and were demonstrating more comfort with novel foods, they still had reservations. I spoke to Heather about incorporating more strategies to make unfamiliar foods more approachable and palatable.

For many kids with food aversions, the prospect of having a nonpreferred or unknown taste or texture in their mouth is the primary hurdle preventing them from consuming new foods. One of the best ways to combat this potentially jarring experience is by consuming a new or nonpreferred food alongside a preferred one. It's a tactic I'm sure we've all put into practice at some point. We strategically employ a sauce, hide a funky green bean in a mound of mashed potatoes or enrobe a foul-tasting medicine in pudding before offering it to our kids. It works. A bite of a new and a preferred food together is less intense than a bite of the new one all on its own, so I encourage the food-skeptical kids I work with to make purposeful pairings whenever possible. I even encourage them to deeply skew the new-to-preferred food ratio. When they're just beginning to explore new tastes, the size or purity of their bite isn't important. The most important thing is their eating something new.

The hiccup that I often encounter when promoting this strategy is that kids with feeding difficulties often dislike eating mixed foods and textures. It's why so many extreme picky eaters gravitate to bland and homogenous foods like chicken nuggets, applesauce, French fries and plain pasta. Helping kids learn to accommodate the more sensory-taxing experience of eating complex or combined textures is one of my goals during our work together, but for many kids, as they're working up to this, there is still a way to meet them in the middle. A simple solution for making the two-food bite technique a kid-friendly experience is to employ a dip.

Dips are wonderful for kids because they're as fun as they are effective. On a functional level, dips mask the taste and texture of foods. They can also ease a child's transition to a new food by helping them know what taste and texture to anticipate and aid with proprioceptive awareness, which would benefit both Chloe and Peter. Finally, dips are fun and versatile.

Even when they use a dip, kids are still getting comfortable with a new food and they are still experiencing its taste and texture. My goal is to help kids learn to comfortably and confidently eat a variety of foods. I recognize the enormity that this transition entails for most children with eating difficulties, which is a big reason why I embrace stepping-stones like dips that can help them overcome their barriers to eating. Of course, I eventually want kids to savor and embrace new foods without the need to cloak them in ketchup or chocolate sauce (yes, I encourage chocolate sauce as well as other indulgent and peculiar alternatives). I also want kids to use dips if they need them because I know that dips can serve as a bridge that will ultimately get them to the place where they are comfortably eating new foods without a buffer.

Chloe and Peter both enjoyed ketchup, applesauce and yogurt, and each had a few other foods that could serve as dips. I explained the benefit of using dips to Heather and encouraged her to serve one of the kids' preferred dips alongside new foods or when she saw them struggling to eat.

Dips would also be useful whenever the kids needed an extra nudge to eat, and I encouraged Heather to invite Chloe and Peter's input on having dips in their meals. I suggested that she could ask the kids to select a dip and let them determine how they wanted it served—on the top, on the side, in a separate dish, etc. I warned her not to resist any unconventional or unappealing requests. It doesn't matter whether a child dips a meatball in mayonnaise or carrots in caramel sauce. Their eating a new food and gaining comfort with unfamiliar tastes and textures are all that matter.

Heather had more positive reports when I next checked in between our scheduled sessions. She was noticing the kids' eating habits evolving. "Chloe has finally tried baked beans and bit into a carrot stick with apple butter on it!" she shared. Throughout our time together, Chloe had been the more resistant of the two kids, so her progress was a tremendous feat for Heather. "I wish we had started earlier," Heather told me. "We could have saved years of stressing."

Beyond the eating accomplishments that continued to accumulate, the kids' attitudes toward mealtimes and food were transforming. Heather told me that they were sitting at the table with more comfort and regularity. Peter was no longer taking it upon himself to seek out dinner alternatives in the kitchen. Even though, due to time constraints, Heather reported that the family wasn't always sharing as many meals as she would like, it had become second nature for them to eat family style and for the kids to serve themselves a portion from every dish on the table. They didn't incorporate a play session every night (some nights the kids seemed too exhausted or the vibe was too frazzled), but Heather didn't ever let them ignore the new foods. They played a game where the kids made guesses about a food's sensory properties—was it heavier or lighter than the chicken nugget? Was it going to feel firm or squishy, cold or warm? Heather noticed that the way Chloe and Peter talked about new food was changing, too. Both seemed to have a more open outlook and their judgments about "good" and "bad," "mine" and "yours" were breaking down.

Additionally, the kids' isolated bites of new foods were slowly translating to meaningful diet expansion. Chloe and Peter weren't yet accustomed to eating every dish they met. Some days they didn't venture from their original diets, but on other days, like the night Peter ate a full portion of fried rice with chicken and vegetables, their days of eating only bland, processed foods seemed far behind them.

Heather was eating with her family and was closer to serving just one meal, but she wasn't entirely there yet. Chloe and Peter still preferred basic foods, like mashed potatoes and orzo with oil, over the more flavorful dishes their parents had, so meals were still a hodgepodge of items, but they had reached a more workable situation. We discussed ways to adapt the kids' basics into more interesting dishes for Heather and her husband, but even as things were, Heather was happy and hopeful of what the future held and believed that Chloe and Peter would continue to make progress. Mealtimes were less stressful and Chloe and Peter both (usually) remained at the table for the entire twenty minutes that they reserved for dinner.

Chloe's intake still seemed to be on a downswing, but Heather resisted pressuring her or even discussing with her how much she ate. Instead, at the end of every meal and snack she gave the kids a warning that the meal was almost over and that the kitchen would be closed until the next scheduled meal. She invited them to eat up if they were still hungry. Sometimes they ate more and sometimes they didn't. She had come to terms with that.

By the time we were finishing up our work together, Heather was pleased with the progress on her goals. She was excited that she could finally incorporate more healthful alternatives into Chloe and Peter's diets, and she was beginning to make headway on her hope to improve their nutritional intake, though she still struggled to accommodate and find overlap with the kids' differing dietary restrictions.

For example, Heather was happy when the kids both ate allergy-friendly blueberry muffins that she made. She hoped to boost them with a protein powder next time. But the kids' food restrictions made it difficult to find an easy way to do so. Peter could share the whey-based protein powder that the rest of the family enjoyed. Only he didn't like it. Heather found an egg protein that Chloe liked, but of course Peter had to steer clear.

As we talked this predicament through, Heather considered where she started and realized this was a problem that she was happy to have. She was no longer constantly struggling with her kids' limited diets and resistance to trying new foods, which meant she could finally shift her focus to optimizing their diets.

Although the process of helping Chloe and Peter learn to welcome new foods was still a work in progress, there was now room for tweaking the areas that Heather had been looking to improve. In just a matter of months, she was looking at a completely different picture, and she was excited for the one she would be facing a few months down the road.

Activity: Discovering Dips

I love using dips to help picky eaters try new foods. Dips are an effective tool because they can mask the taste and texture of foods, which can ease a picky eater's transition to eating something new. I think of them as a fun and tasty stepping-stone that keeps kids grounded in familiarity while also enabling them to branch out to something new.

If your child is already eating dips or any food that could be used to dip (yogurt, soup, applesauce, nut butter, whipped cream), serving dips alongside preferred foods is an easy transition. See some of the suggestions for serving dips on the following pages.

If your child is not currently eating dips, don't turn the page. The strategy can still apply. When introducing new dips to a picky eater, focus on selections that share their favorite flavors. Your child is more likely to enjoy a flavor that is already familiar and comfortable.

Wherever your child is currently at, I recommend embracing this technique with an open mind. Avoid placing limits on your child's dip choice or pairing if it's unconventional. We're not creating a new cuisine or cementing a lifelong habit. In fact, dips should be used as a transitional bridge to facilitate tasting new foods. Once your child is consistently welcoming those, dips can be phased out.

Using Dips at the Table

Build on Preferences: If you're looking to introduce a dip to your child, I recommend sticking to their preferred flavors. Look at your child's favorite foods. Do you notice any patterns? Do they tend to like sweet, salty or spicy foods? Like Peter, who gravitated toward the sweet baked beans, kids are often attracted to particular tastes and will be more likely to welcome a new food that shares their preferred flavors. Incorporating your child's preferences can make using dips more successful.

Invite Input: This is a great opportunity to give a child agency. Let them select their dip and decide where and how they want to use it. I recommend keeping the choice simple. Ask if they prefer one of two options.

Think Outside the Plate: Dips don't need to go on a child's plate alongside their meal. Offer a side plate or tiny dish to hold the dip. Separate containers tend to be really fun, and they're effective for keeping the dip from mixing with other foods on their plate.

Model Pressure-Free Interactions: Model how your child can use a dip. Be playful. Remember, your primary goal is not to encourage eating right away. Dips will help your child acquire the comfort they need to eventually eat a new food. Allow your child to engage at their own pace however they are currently ready to.

Remember to Wean: You don't need to regularly include a dip once your child is comfortable with a new food. You can begin to offer foods they're learning to like on their own and only resort to a dip when your child is struggling or if they request it.

Diving into Dips

Fun activities that don't expressly focus on eating are an ideal entry point for building your child's comfort. Try the activities below or think of your own. Nothing is off-limits!

Use dip as a paint and a novel food as a brush; if the dip is a novel food, consider also using the finger as a brush. Try these activities:

- Apply a dip lipstick.
- Paint your nails using a dip (then lick off the polish!).
- Apply dip tattoos on hands and arms.
- Dot a circle of dip on your nose.
- Dunk a new food in a preferred dip and lick it off like a tasty lollipop.
- Play a game of tic-tac-toe using a dip and a novel food.
- Use dips in a Tastes Test activity (see page 47).
- Drive a novel food through a dip "road."
- Practice writing your name using a dip.
- Make your own dips.
- Pretend the dip is a pool that other foods can "swim" in.

Dips for Every Taste

Sweet

- Ketchup
- Maple syrup
- Honey
- Nutella
- Barbecue sauce
- Jelly
- Chocolate, strawberry or caramel sauce
- Whipped cream
- Applesauce
- Pudding
- Sweetened yogurt

Salty

- Soy sauce
- Gravy
- Steak sauce
- Olive tapenade

Savory

- Cheese sauce
- Mayonnaise
- Hummus
- Alfredo sauce
- Melted butter
- Cream cheese
- Thousand Island or ranch dressing
- Pesto
- Tahini
- Tzatziki sauce
- Tomato sauce
- Guacamole

Spicy

- Cocktail sauce
- Mustard
- Salsa
- Hot sauce

Sour/Tart

- Lemon or lime juice
- Balsamic or red wine vinegar
- Plain yogurt
- Sour cream
- Vinaigrette
- Tartar sauce
- Italian dressing

CHAPTER 7

A Table for One
A Child Who Eats Alone

"It would be nice if we could take a trip as a family without making sure we're within driving distance to a Whole Foods," Lauren confessed the first time we spoke. Her ten-year-old son, Max, was highly particular, not just about the few foods that he ate, but about the specific brands as well. As long as they had access to a kitchen and were near a Whole Foods Market, where most of his preferred items were available, he'd be fine. If not, Max simply wouldn't eat.

It wasn't that he didn't want to eat or that he wasn't hungry enough. Max was unable to bring himself to eat foods that weren't on his safe list. Nonpreferred foods were "gross" and disturbed Max on a visceral level, upsetting him or making him gag. Although he wasn't able to articulate the source of his revulsions, there was no denying their severity. Kids with spectrum disorders, like Max, are prone to inscrutable dislike of certain foods that drives them to maintain extremely restricted diets. Their revulsions to food can be stronger than their desire to eat.

Max was difficult to feed from nearly the moment he was born. He had sensory processing issues and was diagnosed with autism around the age of two. Eating, Lauren shared, had always been a challenge due to Max's aversions to texture, smell and even the appearance of foods. His difficulties actually worsened as he grew older. Max used to enjoy cooking with Lauren. He used to sit with his family for meals. Now he avoided the kitchen, ate alone on the couch and had a meltdown if a nonpreferred food was too close to him. His aversions had become so severe that Max could no longer even tolerate watching others eat.

In typical kid fashion, Max disliked fruits and vegetables. Unlike most kids, however, and even most picky eaters, he actually didn't eat a single one. Overall, Max's diet was fairly uniform. He preferred carbohydrates, especially ones with a homogenous easy-to-manage texture like Cheerios, plain oatmeal, a particular brand of pancake mix, sourdough bread, French fries, Chinese-style white rice and cake. Those formed the foundation of his diet. The only other foods that he ate were his aunt's homemade chicken soup with rice, ice cream and one specific brand each of chicken nuggets and corndogs. Nothing that he ate required much oral dexterity or left much to surprise.

Max grew up with a strong gag reflex that was easily triggered by anything that appeared or smelled not right to him. Although he wasn't as sensitive as he used to be, Max still struggled just looking at or smelling foods outside of his comfort zone, flinching and sometimes still gagging when he encountered them. Because he was extremely loyal not only to particular brands, but also to particular preparations of foods, his aversions extended even to unexpected idiosyncrasies in his preferred foods. For example, pancakes, his breakfast staple, had to be cooked just so—about four inches across and neither too brown nor too light. If they were prepared differently than he was used to, he refused to eat them.

Lauren shared this information with me in our first two conversations. Even though I didn't know Max well yet,

I was familiar with the struggles he was experiencing. The problem wasn't really that he was picky. His food aversions stemmed from severe sensory impairment. It also wasn't that he didn't want to eat a variety of pancakes or more variety in general; it was that the thought of doing so made his skin crawl.

Many extreme picky eaters have at least some sensory involvement that shapes their food preferences or interferes with their ability to accept new foods. Children with impaired sensory integration are known to have abnormal white matter tracts in the parts of their brains that regulate the auditory, visual and tactile systems used to process sensory information. According to experts, these alterations could interfere with proper regulation of sensory stimuli, causing complications in nearly every aspect of their life.[69] It's not surprising, then, that kids with sensory issues experience shortcomings in their behavior, learning, social interactions and even eating habits.

Eating was Max's greatest challenge in part because his sensory dysfunction was more than a complication. It was completely debilitating. There was a part of him that truly couldn't manage consuming or even considering certain foods. On top of that, Max had now been eating the same things in the same way for nearly a decade. Ultimately, his eating habits would be hard to break.

Although they understood that sensory impairments were likely at the root of most of Max's eating aversions, Lauren and Max's dad, Michael, couldn't really comprehend how Max had come to eat fewer than a dozen foods. They wondered if they were to blame.

Most often, feeding difficulties are not a result of parenting, but of a physical problem. That's not to say that parents don't have a role in their child's eating, but research suggests that parents' dispositions, personal eating preferences and even child-rearing practices are not significant contributors to severe picky eating and are not known to impact a child's weight status. A 2010 study following families for nine years, from the time their children were two until they turned eleven, found no significant differences regarding parenting style, pressure to eat and food restriction between the parents of kids who were picky and those who were not.[70] Similarly, researchers exploring maternal eating habits found that while 17 percent of the mothers considered themselves picky, only 4 percent of the children were repeatedly identified as picky between the ages of three to seven, suggesting that even picky parents can't be blamed for a child's selectivity.[71]

Additionally, chronic picky eaters have been found to share a variety of intrinsic impediments, including anxiety, hotheadedness, poor coping mechanisms, elimination problems and physical symptoms such as pain or weakness that might impact their eating.[72,73] Still, we know that parents contribute to a child's eating trajectory insofar as they serve as role models and manage the logistics around their child's eating opportunities. The more a picky eater is allowed to be picky, the more routine those behaviors can become and the more difficult it is then to engage with anything outside of their comfort zone.

As for Max, it was clear to me that he had inherent barriers to eating. There was likely nothing Lauren or Michael could have done to change that. Yet, I did feel that by accommodating idiosyncrasies in an effort to keep Max comfortable and well fed, they had unwittingly fostered his inclination to be selective.

In my early conversations with Lauren it was clear that Max's eating difficulties were deep-rooted and interdependent. I identified aspects of Max's current eating routine that could be optimized to gently increase his exposure to and tolerance of nonpreferred foods. As things were, Max was eating alone and rarely coming into contact with novel foods. These two factors reinforced his aversions, and I believed they needed amending. Additionally, I planned to move his eating from the couch to the kitchen table. We'd then work on techniques to incorporate new foods into his meals and eventually progress to encouraging him to eat new foods and eat alongside his parents.

With a plan in place, we were nearly ready to begin making over Max's mealtime routine, but Lauren and Michael first wanted advice on one other eating quirk that they hadn't yet successfully addressed on their own. Max wasn't independently feeding himself. He only used a utensil to eat cake, ice cream and white rice from his favorite Chinese restaurant. Otherwise, even though he was capable of using a fork and spoon, he didn't. For his daily doses of oatmeal, Cheerios and his aunt's chicken soup, he relied on his family to spoon-feed him. Although he was ten, Max didn't seem to find this problematic. His family, however, knew that it was exceptionally unusual that a ten-year-old hadn't mastered a skill that most do before their second birthday.

I initially thought that Max's insistence for feeding assistance was a behavioral issue. However, after consulting with a colleague and getting to know Max better, I began to wonder if his hang-up with utensils was actually rooted in sensory dysfunction like the rest of his feeding issues seemed to be. The foods that Max ate on his own were relatively tidy, dry solids that were easy to manipulate and didn't crumble when bitten. It was possible that Max didn't feel like he could adequately control a spoon to eat the messier foods in his diet without getting some on his face or dripping them on his shirt. No one loves a mess when they're eating, but most can handle the repercussions when it inevitably happens. Yet Max wasn't in the majority. I suspected that the potential for mess was so threatening that he eliminated the possibility of its occurring.

Helping Max learn to feed himself was a primary goal for Lauren and Michael. Although I agreed that it was peculiar, it wasn't at the top of my list. I did consider that Max's dependence on eating assistance limited his dietary potential, but as things were, Max was only unable to feed himself three foods (granted, this translated to a quarter of his diet). I reasoned that if he could first learn to accept new foods and ultimately expand his diet, he would be less dependent on those three foods and his skill deficit wouldn't be so meaningful. Additionally, Max's sensory system would adapt as he learned to embrace new food. I hoped that once he became more comfortable with eating overall, he might also gain a willingness to feed himself.

The detail that I did feel was necessary to address before starting our interventions was Max's potential nutrient deficits. Max used to be more receptive, and his diet used to be much more diverse. There was a time when he ate chicken, lettuce, black beans, pizza (even with toppings!), hamburgers and several preparations of eggs. And up until a few years ago, he was regularly eating sliced apples, berries and avocado—a small but impressive collection of fruits for a child who no longer tolerated even looking at those foods. Even after he began to drop foods, Lauren and Michael more than once caught him gnawing on a cucumber straight from their garden. They noticed a theme that I've seen repeated throughout the picky eater population. Eating evolves, but not in the desired direction. Parents often share a history of their child's dwindling food acceptance and progressively narrow diet that inspires them to seek support.

By the time Lauren and Michael did so, Max had restricted his diet to the point that it lacked vibrancy. Everything that he ate was a carbohydrate in a pale shade of white or brown. High-starch, monochromatic, low-variety diets are common among extreme picky eaters, so much so that it's become an infamous eating pattern associated with the population. Picky eaters aren't born attracted to these foods. Instead, they find comfort in their consistency. Even the most basic vegetables, like carrots, that are sweet and lack seeds or skin, have variations in their color, texture, taste and overall look. These unexpected inconsistencies irk picky eaters, which is why most gravitate to simple packaged foods.

Max found comfort in his beige diet, but I worried it did not provide him with the breadth of nutrition that he needed. He seemed to be consuming ample calories to support his growth and sustain his energy; however, because he eschewed fruits and vegetables, which house nutrients that are otherwise available only in a multivitamin, and because he was not taking any supplements, it was possible that he was missing out on essential vitamins and minerals.

Micronutrient deficiencies not only impact health and growth but can also contribute to an array of more general impairments, including irritability, decreased attention, lethargy, appetite loss and taste changes. These symptoms can interfere with a child's ability to eat a balanced meal, perpetuating an unfortunate cycle that extreme picky eaters can't escape. A lackluster diet can cause nutrient deficiencies, contributing to impaired appetite, energy and attention, ultimately resulting in diminished mealtime stamina and even more food refusal, which further fuels the dilemma.

It was impossible to definitively link Max's history of irritable outbursts and idiosyncratic food preferences with deficient vitamin and mineral levels, but that didn't mean there was no benefit to supplementing his diet. Therefore, before we set out to help Max learn to embrace a greater variety of foods, I recommended Lauren start supplementing his diet with a flavorless powdered multivitamin that she could mix into his almond milk or pancakes without his knowing.

This caught Lauren off guard at first. She knew that I was not a proponent of sneaking more nutritious foods into a picky eater's favorites. I explained that I saw a distinction. Hiding foods—like pureeing vegetables into a sauce—doesn't provide kids with the opportunity to learn to accept nutritious foods on their own terms, and can often cause them to have distrust of caregivers, an enhanced fear of unfamiliar foods and a further distaste for the hidden food.[74] Discovering an unexpected multivitamin mixed into a favorite dish could be equally as traumatic for an unsuspecting child; however, the potential benefits of correcting impaired nutrient levels are often, in my opinion, worth attempting. Max wouldn't accept a traditional vitamin and wouldn't eat his favorite foods if he knew they were mixed with a powder. Supplementing without his knowledge was our only option.

After Lauren started Max on the vitamin, she didn't notice a discernable difference in his behavior or general well-being, but that didn't mean it wasn't working. I warned Lauren not to expect the multivitamin to have a dramatic effect. It can take months for vitamin deficiencies to correct, and it was also possible that there would be no obvious improvement at all. I wanted to ensure that Max was getting the nutrition that he needed, and vitamin supplementation was the most efficient way to achieve that.

In our first conversation, before we addressed Lauren and Michael's concerns about Max's feeding skills and mine about his potential vitamin deficiencies, Lauren had said that her ultimate goal was to be able to share meals as a family. I took this to mean more broadly that she wanted Max to be comfortable eating with others in social situations, whether it was with his parents at home, in a restaurant, with a friend, at school or on vacation. I was hopeful that Max would eventually get to that point, but transitioning to family meals in his case was not as simple or neat as it sounded.

Because Max was eating a handful of foods in isolation and couldn't even tolerate the thought or sight of nonpreferred foods, the transition would not be as straightforward as sitting Max down at the kitchen table with his parents. I broke down Max's journey from where he was to where Lauren wanted him to be into steps. The first would be learning to eat alone at the table where the family ate their meals instead of on the couch. I saw the table as the springboard to future steps that he would have to accomplish. Once he was at the table, we'd bring in the next components of a family meal: first new foods, then his family members. Each step of this journey would build on the other, creating a foundation of support that would allow Max's eating habits to evolve comfortably. I shared this bird's-eye view of the plan for Max with Lauren and Michael at the end of our first session.

In our next session, a week later, we began the first and simplest step of the intervention: transitioning Max's meals to the kitchen table where the family ate. Its simplicity was only part of why I selected this adjustment as our first step. Max was in the habit of eating his meals on the couch, often with the television on. I suspected that the couch and TV both took Max's attention away from eating, making it easier for him to do so more comfortably.

Max's comfort was at the forefront of my mind, but it was important for him to learn to be present while eating, not just for its own sake but also as a way to help him move forward. In order to grow comfortable being around new foods, Max first needed to be present during exposures to new foods. He needed to see their colors and shapes, get to know their smells and textures and hear the noises they made when eaten. If we could first get him more focused on his own food, the transition to interacting with other foods would be less jarring.

Eating at the family's large distraction-free kitchen table had other perks. First, eating there would set the stage for shared family-style meals. Second, the physical support Max would gain from sitting at the table might have the added benefit of helping him feel he could eat independently.

I talked to Lauren and Michael about the potential influence of a positive, relaxed and distraction-free eating environment in fostering healthy eating habits. It was important for Max to eat at a table that was uncluttered and comfortable, which for him meant a table free of superfluous stimuli like fragrant flowers, overly bright lights, noisy cutlery and activity in the kitchen while he was eating.

Before moving Max's meals, Michael spoke to him about the plan to work with me and about his and Lauren's hopes for Max's eating. Max seemed to understand his parents' motivations on a logical level. He wanted those things, too, he said. Yet he was not receptive when Michael shared that mealtimes would begin to look different than he was used to. We were therefore all happily surprised when Max didn't protest to moving his meals to the table.

I met with Lauren and Michael again just two weeks after we decided to introduce Max to meals at the table. By then, that's where Max was eating all of his meals. Not every meal was seamless, though. Lauren told me that Max was frequently struggling to stay seated for the duration of his meal, and he often requested to turn on the TV. She wanted to know if it was okay to compromise and let Max eat with an iPad to help him stay seated on the days he struggled to focus. I advised against it.

As with everything that Max was about to encounter, eating at the table was a tremendous departure from what he knew. Even though the scenery was not so significantly different—the kitchen table was not far from the living room; you could see each when sitting at the other—the principle effect was meaningful. It signaled that Max's comfortable routine was in jeopardy.

I actually thought that Max's transition seemed perfectly natural. I didn't expect it to be seamless. Eating without the TV was likely challenging both Max's attention span and his sensory system and he was reacting accordingly. That was okay. He needed to learn to eat without a crutch. Reintroducing a screen at mealtimes would stall Max's progress, so I advised against it. We didn't want to encourage another habit that we would eventually want to break. The easier we could make the process for Max, the better he would feel about it and the less resistant he would be to future adjustments.

Now that Max was accustomed to eating his meals at the table, we shifted the focus of our efforts to introducing new foods. My plan was to acclimate Max to eating in the proximity of nonpreferred foods. Once he tolerated being around them, we could then address his learning to eat them and his learning to eat with others. To get started, I offered Lauren and Michael one simple, foundational guideline: add a small portion of one novel food to Max's meals.

They could, for example, serve a side of fruit alongside a plate of fries and chicken nuggets, but because Max was hypersensitive and had a history of severe aversions to non-preferred food, I didn't anticipate that they could simply set a new food on the table and expect him to be okay with it. I always recommend starting with small portions to minimize a child's overwhelm, and I had a feeling doing so would be extra important for Max.

I advised Lauren and Michael to begin with a serving size that was no larger than a grain of rice. The goal of the tiny portion was for Max to be comfortable enough that he could sit with the food and eventually taste it. Repeated tasting, not the size of the taste, seems to be the most significant factor in the development of preferences. Therefore, the only detail that mattered was that the portion size was manageable for Max.

Once Max was able to tolerate being around the new food and worked up to tasting it, Lauren and Michael could increase the bite size, moving first to a serving the size of a dried bean, then a raspberry and so forth, until Max was eating an age-appropriate portion.

Similarly, rather than asking Max to tolerate new foods directly on his plate, which would be a significant departure from what he was used to, I suggested Lauren provide him with a side plate. The separate plate would further reinforce a distinction between these new foods and the staples that created the rest of his meal, but Max already knew that new foods were different. I felt Max would appreciate the buffer that a separate plate allowed. I told Lauren to let him know that he could move it away if the proximity was overwhelming. Even though this would add distance between Max and the new foods, moving the plate would actually give Max a short but valuable interaction with the novel foods.

To further ease Max's transition and to increase the likelihood that he would feel comfortable enough to eventually eat the new foods he encountered at mealtimes, Lauren and I created a strategic bank of five new foods that she should focus on. My aim was to acclimate Max to new experiences, not to alienate him. We therefore selected a combination of foods that Max used to eat as well as new ones that shared his preferred sensory properties.

Apples, plain pasta, potatoes, eggs and cucumber made the first cut. In addition to being nutritious foods that would greatly improve the quality of Max's diet, eggs, cucumber and apples were familiar foods that Max used to eat. I selected the two other foods, plain pasta and potatoes, because of their sensory properties. Both are starchy, bland and beige. Additionally, they weren't completely novel. Max had observed the rest of his family eating noodles in his aunt's chicken soup, and Max regularly ate potatoes as French fries and potato chips.

I encouraged Lauren to experiment with the presentation of the goal foods. Try the cucumbers cut into spears, coins, chunks or tiny pieces, I told her. Mash cooked potatoes with some soup broth or serve them in strips like fries. We didn't know which style would appeal to Max, and I wanted to present him with as many opportunities to succeed as possible. Additionally, encountering the variety of presentations would help Max get used to eating foods that are different and reduce the likelihood that he would get locked into expecting the new foods to be prepared in certain ways.

Lauren and I checked in frequently over the next few weeks as she focused on incorporating new foods into Max's mealtimes. She told me that Max didn't initially respond as dramatically to the nonpreferred foods as she had anticipated. The first couple of times that he sat down to eat with a plate of new foods beside him, he appeared upset, but not viscerally uncomfortable. Instead of gagging or refusing to sit, he was simply negative. He said that the eggs looked like barf. He didn't want to be near them. The apple, cucumbers, pasta and potatoes were also gross, nasty or disgusting. Though Max tolerated the foods from a sensory perspective, he made it clear that he did not want to be around them.

After two more weeks of protesting the addition of "gross" new foods on the table, Max started to become increasingly distraught at mealtimes. More than once Lauren told me that at dinner Max became more riled up than she had ever seen him. He was regularly irritable, recalcitrant and rude, seemingly furious about having to sit near even the tiny portions of new foods. Lauren wasn't sure how to handle his outbursts in the context of their new routine. She didn't want to upset Max further, but would there ever be a change if she didn't follow through?

Lauren and Michael told me that since introducing new foods they felt like they were constantly having to manage Max's behavior and that instead of enjoying his progress, they were ruining their relationship with him. Negotiating his unpleasantness, knowing when to push him and when to tend to his tantrums, proved to be Lauren's biggest struggle as we moved forward. She found his dramatic behavior difficult to contend with and even harder to decipher. Was Max rebelling or was it a sign that his sensory system was under attack?

I interpreted Max's change in behavior as an indication that we were pushing him too far or too quickly, or both. Rather than abandon our plan, I sought to make the task more manageable for him. I advised Lauren and Michael to stick with rice-sized pieces of new foods and told them to reinforce that, though the foods weren't going anywhere, Max didn't have to eat them. Additionally, I wanted to meet with Max in person to offer him coping mechanisms that would help him more comfortably endure mealtimes at home as well as have comfortable food experiences in the future. Lauren and I scheduled a session with Max for the following week.

I had seen videos of Max eating before, but this was my first time meeting him. Despite his deep-rooted struggles to eat, Max wasn't particularly thin. Although he had no trouble maintaining attention throughout our conversation, he was reserved, and it was clear that he would have preferred to have been doing something else.

I started by explaining to Max that his body might have strong reactions to encountering new foods. His reactions wouldn't be permanent or harmful. In fact, they were helpful. "They're letting you know that you need more time getting to know these foods," I told him, explaining that I could teach him tricks to manage the uncomfortable responses so he could learn to like new foods and eventually share meals with his friends and family. He was open to exploring some of these strategies.

I started with my favorite strategy, hoping that Max would like it, too. "If there's a new food that you are ready to taste," I told him, "you might take a bite and realize it doesn't taste right to your body. You can just spit it out into your napkin if you change your mind. Or, you could immediately follow it with a taste of a preferred food or beverage. You could even eat a favorite and new food together. That way, the flavor and texture of the preferred food would mask those of the new one."

Those sounded like good tips to Max, but he wasn't yet at the point where he was tasting new foods during his meals. Other barriers were standing in his way. I advised him to push his new food plate away from his immediate space if he felt uncomfortable having it nearby. He could even cover it with a napkin. If he was struggling with smells of new foods, I recommended that he cover serving dishes to trap the smell. He could even ask his parents to bring a fan into the kitchen or light a candle to mask an unpleasant smell. I made a note to tell Lauren and Michael that serving foods at room temperature instead of hot was also a great trick to mute the intensity of their aroma. Finally, I encouraged Max to pay attention to what his body was telling him as he encountered new foods and to think of his own ways to address its needs.

Max only had a week to put the new strategies into practice before I met with the family again for a fourth session. Lauren and Michael reported that since I had met with Max, meals had been calmer. Instead of protesting the presence of new foods, Max was opting to push his side plate far down the table or cover it up with a napkin.

Sensing some disappointment from Lauren and Michael in terms of Max's progress, I reminded them that the techniques Max was employing were not cop-outs. I didn't see them as setbacks, and I encouraged them to continue suggesting them to Max when he struggled. The adjustments were stepping-stones, a solution for meeting Max in the middle and helping him get from where he was to where he needed to go.

Lauren and Michael were not reassured. "When I think about where we were weeks ago, things are better, but I keep wishing he were further along," Lauren shared with me. She lamented that Max was not yet actively engaging with new foods despite my conversation with him last week and despite the fact that she was presenting him with daily opportunities to do so. She was frustrated, too, that Max wasn't receptive even to foods she thought would go over well.

Max had said on a few occasions that he liked the way his aunt's pasta sauce smelled. Lauren thought it was a good idea to offer him a drop of sauce on his side plate, but Max objected when it was closer than an arm's length away. When Lauren reminded him that he didn't have to eat it and suggested that he engage with it in a fun way, by smelling it or dipping a French fry in it, he not so politely declined.

I understood Lauren's frustration. She had implemented significant changes in spite of Max's defiance. Her efforts seemed futile. But we weren't done yet. I still had more approaches I wanted to address with Lauren and Michael. Importantly, I also had more that I wanted to share with Max.

We set aside a few minutes at the start of our fourth session for another short conversation with Max. Now that he had tools to help him engage comfortably with new foods, I wanted him to understand that learning to do so was a process. Max was just at the beginning and there was no expectation that he would jump immediately from meeting new foods to eating them. "Not only is the transition hard," I told him, "but there are actually many steps in between those two markers."

I walked Max through Toomey's Steps to Eating, letting him know that if he wasn't ready to eat yet, there were a number of alternatives for how he could engage with a new food, like talking about how it looked or smelled, or touching it with a utensil to see whether it was soft or hard. I shared, too, about the likelihood that his transition wouldn't be instantaneous and that I hoped he'd stick with it anyway. Scientists, I told him, have found that people often need to taste a food more than ten times before their taste buds adjust to the new experience and they're actually comfortable eating it. I warned him that older kids and kids with barriers to eating might need to double or triple that number. Max took this in with no questions or reservations and went off on his own while I finished speaking with Lauren and Michael.

Because Lauren was concerned and Max seemed to need a lot of time to warm up to new foods at the table, I wanted to explore inviting ways we could encourage him to independently interact with more foods outside of mealtimes. So far, he was comfortable only tolerating them nearby. This was a big development for him. Still, I thought he would benefit from a different approach to moving along the Steps to Eating.

I was delighted to learn that Max actually had a positive history of participating in both of my preferred means of engaging with food outside of mealtimes: cooking and gardening. As a young child, he had enjoyed cooking and baking alongside Lauren. Although Max was particular about the recipes he'd help with and usually didn't eat the foods he helped prepare, his sensory aversions had seemed to evaporate when he was involved with a recipe. Similarly, when he was younger, the garden had been a place where Max seemed free to try, or at the least touch, foods that he otherwise found unappealing. He seemed to derive the same sense of comfortable satisfaction tending to a growing plant as he did from preparing a recipe.

Max had fallen out of the habit of both activities. Lauren and Michael couldn't pinpoint why. Maybe Max had just gotten older, maybe his sensory aversions had become more severe or maybe it was a combination of both. Regardless of the reason for Max's departure from the kitchen and garden, I hoped that he would be able to rekindle his attraction to the activities. Both offer rich opportunities that could diminish his sensory defensiveness and reverse his resistance to encountering new foods.

Additionally, both activities could increase Max's willingness to eat new foods. Children who cook regularly are more likely to try novel foods and eat more vegetables than those who don't.[75] Similarly, kids are more likely to eat vegetables that they grow. Middle schoolers who participated in garden-based activities that included growing, taste testing and preparing fruit- and vegetable-based dishes ate more fruits and vegetables—and also expressed higher enjoyment of them—than kids who did not complete the activities.[76] Studies suggest that the benefits of engaging in these activities are long lasting. College students who gardened as kids have been found to eat more fruits and vegetables than their peers who had never gardened.[77]

So, a little over a month into our time together, after Max talked the plan over with his parents, he agreed to get back into the garden. Max happily selected plants—tomatoes, strawberries, cucumbers and carrots, as well as an array of herbs—for Lauren to cook with.

Over the course of the next few weeks, Lauren and Michael told me that Max liked tending to his growing plants and was eager to check their progress every few days. Lauren and Michael never discussed whether Max had any intentions of eating his future harvest. If he sensed any pressure, we knew he might lose interest. Even if he never ate what he grew, he was still gaining a multitude of other benefits including sensory exposure, responsibility and patience.

When left on his own, Max did eventually come to enjoy eating the fruits of his labor. Lauren contacted me a few weeks after we finished our regular meetings to share that she had spotted Max snacking on cherry tomatoes in the garden. She started including them in his rotation of new foods at mealtimes and Max was actually eating them!

While Max was honing his green thumb, Lauren began inviting him into the kitchen with her on the weekends, and Max's aunt offered to teach him how to make her signature sauce and soup.

Max resisted at first, but I loved Lauren and Max's aunt's approach to cooking with him. Their invitation was casual and organic, free of pressure or ulterior motive. This no-strings approach was crucial for Max. If he sensed his participation was a requirement or that there were certain expectations for his behavior, he'd be turned off. The kitchen was no longer a comfortable place for him due to the barrage of sensory stimuli. I told Lauren to remind Max of the techniques I had shared with him a few weeks ago to make the experiences easier, and I provided Lauren with additional tips. Max could wear gloves so he wouldn't have to touch anything directly, use extra-long utensils so he wouldn't have to get too close to anything and keep a spare towel close by so he could wipe off his hands as needed. I also suggested trying basic recipes that didn't require too much hands-on time or smell too strongly, such as salad with dressing or baked goods.

After two weeks of invitations, Max did eventually join his family in the kitchen, helping with whatever they were preparing. Once he became comfortable, I spoke with Lauren about incorporating intentional activities to help break down his rigid eating habits.

Max was highly particular about the specific preparation of most of the foods he ate. For example, he didn't like pancakes or soup *in general*; he liked *one specific* variation of each. Comfortable eaters often don't have problems handling variability in their food. That sort of rigidity, however, is a hallmark of many extreme picky eaters. Kids who struggle to eat often focus on minute details about their foods to the point that it holds them back from eating. I knew that we couldn't simply offer Max variations on his favorites and expect him to eat them. But I hoped that he might feel differently if he was the one responsible for making the changes. My goal wasn't for Max to learn to eat around stray vegetables in his soup or to like a different brand of pancake mix. Instead, I hoped learning to tolerate these changes would translate to his becoming more flexible with food overall. Involving him in making small alterations to the texture, taste or appearance of his preferred foods could help him understand that even with some minor changes, the essence of his preferred foods was not changing, that his food was still the same even though one minor characteristic was different.

I provided Lauren with some examples of how to help Max make some tweaks to his foods, and within the next few days she suggested that Max join her making pancakes. Lauren showed him how to make them as he liked and then offered some of the options that we had discussed: they could add a bit of food dye or extra liquid, mix in chocolate chips, spoon the batter into bigger circles or cut his usual circles into shapes using a cookie cutter. When he was ready to be more adventurous, Max could incorporate fruit or oats or add some spices like cinnamon to change the flavor.

Max took to the pancake project, opting to use a cookie cutter to create new shapes from his standard pancakes. Lauren reminded Max that he didn't have to eat. As with most of the strategies, it took Max some time to work up to eating the new presentation. Eventually, he did, though. After about a week of cookie cutting his pancakes, Max ate one in a star shape, the first time in Lauren didn't remember how long that he didn't require circles.

Even more significant in Lauren and Michael's eyes was the following anecdote: One afternoon as Lauren was preparing dinner, she looked over to the table to find Max eating Cheerios with a spoon all on his own. He hadn't even asked for help. "This is HUGE," Lauren shared with me over email.

With these big accomplishments, I felt confident that Max was moving in the right direction, but Lauren and Michael were still underwhelmed by his progress so far. They felt that all of their efforts weren't translating to noticeable improvements in Max's daily intake.

I tried to help them see that while it might be slow and though it certainly wasn't flashy, Max was improving in significant ways. Since starting to work together around two months ago, Max had learned how to more comfortably handle being around nonpreferred foods. Additionally, his flexibility with the pancakes had so much potential. I saw it as a step toward a future in which Max could order pancakes at a restaurant or enjoy them at a friend's house. If he continued to make similar advancements, he would no longer be bound to his ultra-specific foods. This time I reminded Lauren and Michael about the likely slow path Max was embarking on. I hoped they could recognize and celebrate the small accomplishments Max would make as he worked his way to the ultimate goal of eating.

Due to Max's growing tolerance and engagement with new foods, at our next session I recommended finally attempting shared meals. Witnessing others eat had historically made Max cringe. It stood in the way of his eating lunch with his friends at school and precluded him from casually encountering novel foods.

My homework for Lauren and Michael was to begin eating together as a family as often as possible. Any meal, any time of day. Though Lauren and Michael had been craving having family meals for years, it proved to be harder than they had anticipated. They tried sharing breakfast first. Lauren and Michael had yogurt and Max had star-shaped pancakes with an apple slice on the side. Lauren and Michael told me that Max tolerated the meal, but with the company of both of his parents and their meals, he failed to eat as well as usual. Max's paltry intake didn't seem sustainable to them given that he didn't eat lunch at school, so after two attempts of poor intake, they switched their focus to dinner.

After three weeks of trying to come together in the evening, Lauren and Michael were disappointed to share that the family had only eaten as a threesome three times. They cited challenges with their work schedules. More often, Max ate alone or with only one parent. I assured Lauren and Michael that even their one-on-one meals with Max offered the same benefits of behavior modeling and new food exposure as eating all together would. Yet these sorts of meals weren't what Lauren and Michael had been envisioning, and it was clear that they felt badly about their inability to eat together more often.

"Do people actually do this?" Lauren kept asking me. She wondered whether families with two working parents were really eating dinner together during the week. "If they are, can you share their secrets?"

There's a difference between what's ideal and what's real, I explained to Lauren and Michael the night they reported their disappointment of having only three shared meals in three weeks. I had recommended they eat together as often as possible, ideally once per day. This ideal, unfortunately, wasn't realistic for their family at this time. I was okay with that and I wanted them to be, too.

I reminded them that they were still putting in a lot of work helping Max. Yes, I believed shared meals were important. Yes, the more often they ate together, the easier it would become for Max to tolerate the stressors of eating among both company and a variety of foods, the more incentive he would have to branch out and the faster he would see progress. But family meals were just one piece in the larger puzzle of factors that would help Max learn to welcome new foods. I wanted them to continue trying, but a failure to come together regularly was not going to sabotage Max's progress.

Even as Lauren and Michael struggled with their inability to eat together as a family, they continued exposing Max to new foods, encouraging him to engage and promoting his time in the garden and kitchen. Over the next few weeks, Max began to demonstrate signs of growth.

Lauren and Michael were shocked, though not thrilled (I was), to learn that Max ate a bagel with cream cheese and a hot dog one day while out with a friend. As healthy eaters, Lauren and Michael had been hoping to fill Max's diet with more nutritious foods. I urged them not to let their expectations cloud the significance of Max's accomplishment. Max's decision to eat a new food was a big deal. It didn't matter exactly what new food he ate. It didn't matter that the bagel was starchy and beige like every one of his safe foods or that the hot dog was essentially a corndog in disguise. His eating foods that weren't exactly like his preferred ones was what mattered. The cream cheese especially signified Max's growing flexibility and openness with food. It was a significant first step on a long journey that would ultimately culminate in a number of new and diverse eating experiences.

Even with my cheerleading and reminders, after more than three months of effort, Lauren and Michael were struggling to remain optimistic. In many ways, when we reached the end of our initial time together, it looked like Max was still the same severely selective eater he was four months prior. He was still eating only a dozen foods and he was still unable to share the family meal. But, in even more ways, he had grown tremendously. Max was now eating more often with his family and friends, he tolerated novel foods in his personal space, he was eating cereal on his own and, as for his preferred foods, he was no longer as rigid about their presentation.

Progress doesn't always look the way we expect or hope. Lauren and Michael had reached out to me looking to transform their picky eater. To them, that meant seeing more variety and nutrition in Max's diet and eating as a family at home, in restaurants and on vacation. Though they recognized how far Max had come, Lauren and Michael ached for normalcy, and they felt like they deserved it given how dedicated they had been to Max's transformation.

"Normal" eating doesn't always look the way we expect. To me it doesn't mean eating specific foods or eating them in specific places. Instead, normalcy is being able to let one's desires and preferences, not visceral aversions, govern food choices. Therefore, I don't think it's helpful to hope for "normalcy" or to compare one's own child to others. Parents will find more joy in their lives when they focus on the small steps that signify their child's growing flexibility with food instead of regretting ideals they don't currently have. Lauren and Michael did deserve to see the improvements in their son's eating that they were envisioning. Instead of focusing myopically on these outcomes, I hoped that they would soon realize that Max was working his way there in his own time.

When Lauren and I discussed whether it made sense to continue our work together, she was still trying to reconcile where they were in the process, all that she had done and where she wanted to go. I believed she had the foundation in place to support Max, but I understood that Max's eating was still a work in progress. As we decided to put a hold on our work together, I assured her that the discrepancy she was seeing between her and Michael's effort and their goals was not a result of their not doing enough or of our not doing the right things for Max. I believed time was the only missing ingredient.

If a child's eating issues have been incubating since birth to the day I start seeing them, it's unrealistic to expect progress after only a few sessions or even a few months.

In my experience, families often anticipate immediate and drastic results as soon as they start making changes to what and how they feed their child. Progress feels like it should be inevitable, if for no other reason than as payoff for their hard work. One of the most difficult parts of my job is communicating to parents that their child's transformation will be a long journey. Although no one likes to hear it, some severe picky eaters take years to make meaningful progress. Throughout those years, they will still experience accomplishments—some sporadic, some monumental, others more mundane. The bottom line is that a child with extreme picky eating habits needs a long time to develop a new relationship with food.

Nobody can dictate or guarantee the rate or degree of progress. In my work, I strive to provide families and children with the resources to embark on a path that will ultimately lead to the transformations they desire. In the meantime, I hope to help parents see that every step along that path is one that makes eating more comfortable for their child.

Lauren, Michael and Max were well on their way to where they wanted to go. Although the route wasn't looking like the one Lauren and Michael had hoped for, I urged them to stick with it. They had the tools they needed to get to where they wanted to go. Patience and persistence were the only other requirements needed to help them on their way.

Activity: Comfortable Cooking with a Timid Eater

The kitchen is often the last place a skeptical eater wants to be. They've learned that it can be a sensory danger zone and have become conditioned to avoid the place where food originates. But children are more likely to eat a food when they are involved in its preparation.

Cooking is meant to be fun. Try not to overcomplicate it, and don't let concerns about the mess or the quality of the final product hold you back. Follow these guidelines to make cooking as approachable and beneficial as possible.

How to Get Started

Preparing food, like eating, engages all of the senses. That's part of why it's such a valuable activity. But the sensory exposures can be overwhelming for those with delicate systems. If your child is hesitant to engage with food for a sensory or any other reason, consider easing them into their kitchen experiences by including them in some less intimidating activities, such as organizing the pantry, reading a recipe or gathering ingredients. These can be meaningful stepping-stones to hands-on cooking activities.

When your child is ready to begin cooking, make any necessary adaptations to set them up for success. Consider some of the following ideas to best accommodate your child's sensitivities:

If your child is sensitive to noise:

- Use rubber utensils and plastic bowls that clang less than metal ones.

- Avoid recipes that call for noisy appliances.
- Use a visual timer instead of an audible one.
- Avoid stovetop recipes that may sizzle and pop.

If your child is sensitive to scent:
- Begin with recipes like salad dressing, pesto, dips, salads and sandwiches that don't require heat.
- Avoid cooking with aromatics like garlic and onion.
- Enlist their help preparing the dough or batter for a baked good.

If your child is sensitive to tactile experiences:
- Offer thin medical gloves for handling food.
- Stash a cloth or towel within reach to wipe dirty hands.
- Offer long utensils that provide a safe distance from food.
- Let them do the measuring and mixing.

If your child is sensitive to light:
- Adjust the lighting so it's comfortable for them.
- Be aware of any flashing clocks or bright lights from electronics.

Start Simply
If your child is hesitant to touch food, begin with easy tasks. Some fun introductory activities include:

- Tearing herbs or lettuces
- Cutting soft produce
- Washing produce and dishes
- Collecting ingredients
- Lining muffin tins
- Greasing a pan
- Measuring and mixing
- Setting the timer

Taste as You Go

Tasting is a vital part of cooking—and it's a big reason why I love cooking with children who are hesitant to taste new foods at the table. Keep tiny tasting spoons within reach so it's easy to take a manageable taste. If your child usually isn't a fan of eating new foods, don't emphasize "taking a taste." Instead, pose the question, "What else do we need to add to make this recipe delicious?" Sampling and then adjusting until food tastes right is a wonderful opportunity to establish a positive relationship with food while exploring new flavors.

Avoid Mealtime Prep

Instead of bringing your child into meal prep, carve out some time to be in the kitchen between meals so your child can learn the ropes without the risk of interfering with a meal. Some parents like cooking with their kids after a meal. That way, kids are already fed and happy, and the kitchen is already messy.

Age-Appropriate Cooking Activities
Under 3 Years
- Pouring premeasured items into a bowl
- Tearing greens and herbs
- Using cookie and biscuit cutters
- Washing vegetables
- Measuring ingredients
- Stirring ingredients
- Mashing with a fork or potato masher

Ages 3 to 5
- Cutting soft ingredients
- Mixing
- Spreading (butter, icing, etc.)
- Breading and flouring

- Kneading, rolling and cutting dough
- Peeling hard-boiled eggs and citrus

Ages 5 to 7
- Cutting soft and firm ingredients
- Whisking
- Grating vegetables or cheese
- Cracking eggs
- Cutting with scissors

Ages 8 and Older
- Using a handheld mixer
- Boiling eggs and pasta
- Using the stove with supervision
- Using a peeler
- Making salad dressing

Recipe Ideas for Skeptical Eaters
- Salad dressing in a jar
- Pizza
- Pancakes
- Nachos
- Mashed potatoes
- Skewers with fruits, veggies, meat, cheese, etc.
- Salsa
- Fruit salad in a jar
- Yogurt parfaits
- Salad
- Muffins
- Smoothies
- Overnight oats

Part 2

INTERVENTION PLANS

Ten Tips for Successfully Introducing New Foods

When implementing the intervention plans in this part of the book, keep the following ten tips in mind. I will elaborate on many of them in the upcoming pages; however, they're important guidelines to help you stay on track and ensure that you are supporting your child in their journey of learning to like new foods.

1. Serve one new food at every meal and every snack.

2. Always provide at least one item that your child almost always eats at every meal.

3. Limit eating and drinking (except for water) between meals.

4. Model the eating behavior you'd like your child to demonstrate.

5. Outside of shared meals, present only one new food at a time.

6. Don't pressure your child to eat.

7. Continue to serve a food even if your child doesn't eat it at first.

8. Be patient.

9. Be realistic with your expectations and offerings.

10. Don't obsess over each individual meal or food. If you are regularly exposing your child to new food, you are doing a fantastic job.

A Quick Note on Implementing Change

On average, it can take anywhere from eighteen to two hundred days for an individual to form a new habit.[78] That's why I don't recommend introducing the following suggestions all at once. Instead, take them one at a time. I recommend first reading through the intervention plans, pinpointing a logical place to start and then giving yourself a few days to get used to it.

I usually recommend that my clients try a new routine for a minimum of three days before adding on a new one, but as you've seen in the case studies, change often takes more time than that. It's the lesson I share with and constantly repeat to every family I work with. Give yourself time and be patient as you move forward. Please don't bite off more than you can chew, and please don't give up after just one day or even one week of trying!

CHAPTER 8

What Meals Should Look Like

When first looking to improve extreme picky eating, start with mealtimes. Mealtimes form the foundation of what and how a child eats. No attempt to improve your child's eating will be as successful as it could be if the environment in which they are eating and meeting new foods is not supportive.

The goal is for your family to enjoy positive meals together that provide your selective eater with the opportunity to encounter new foods in a safe and pressure-free setting. If you're like most of the families I've met, you've been craving meals like these for years. It's putting these desires into practice that seems impossible.

Transforming mealtimes starts with addressing the details that go into feeding your family. I recommend using Ellyn Satter's Division of Responsibility (DOR) as a framework for introducing more productive and peaceful meals in your home. The DOR, which is recognized as a best practice by the Academy of Nutrition and Dietetics and the American Academy of Pediatrics, is a model that outlines the parent and child roles in feeding and eating.

Division of Responsibility for Feeding

According to the DOR, parents take leadership with the *what, when* and *where* of feeding. Children are responsible for *whether* and *how much* they want to eat what the parent provides. Before we get to specifics about the *what, when* and *where* of feeding, it's important to know why this model works and what it seeks to help you accomplish.

Underlying these mealtime roles is the idea that structure, support and mutual trust allow children to develop a positive, healthy relationship with food while also setting them up to learn to eat a variety of foods and behave appropriately at mealtimes. By creating a supportive mealtime environment, you are providing the foundation that your child needs to eat well and meet their nutritional needs. Essentially, when caregivers do their job with feeding, it allows children to do their job with eating.

If you're raising an extremely selective eater, this approach may initially sound impractical and completely irrelevant to your current situation, but the DOR is known to support kids of all ages and at all stages on the picky eating spectrum. You have even seen this to be true in the case studies shared in Part 1 of this book. Because extreme picky eaters already have negative associations with new foods and eating, they might actually benefit the most from this framework, which shows them that they have control over their food and that eating can be fun.

At the heart of the DOR is eliminating pressure associated with eating. Because parents are trusting their child to dictate *whether* and *how much* they are eating, there is no room for pressure tactics or self-imposed pressure regarding your child's eating habits. When there is no pressure to eat and kids are left to engage with food however they are ready to, they can relax and feel comfortable around food, which opens the door for trust and exploration.

Following the DOR allows you to let go of your expectations about how meals go and about which and how much of the provided foods your child eats. It can therefore ease much of the anxiety that you feel when feeding your child. Remember, a supportive environment at meals helps your child learn healthy and nutritious eating habits.

Action Plan: Consider any barriers you have to following the DOR. If this framework is new, find time to discuss it with your family. When talking with your child, emphasize that they will have complete control in deciding how much they want to eat at meals and snacks.

Where to Eat

Choose a table in your home to eat at consistently. Sticking to a consistent location is crucial, but it is just as important to avoid eating in areas that have other purposes, such as the couch. To create an environment that facilitates eating, clear all clutter and eliminate distractions from your designated eating location. This means turning off the television and tablets and keeping favorite toys and other temptations out of sight. Distractions might help your child sit at the table more comfortably in the moment, but they ultimately hinder their learning to overcome their barriers to eating.

If your child is not yet ready to sit at the table for meals, begin by taking incremental steps that move them away from where they are currently comfortable and closer to the dining table. For example, if your child is currently eating meals alone in their room and is not comfortable eating at a kitchen table, have them first acclimate to eating at a table in their room. As they acclimate to eating at the table, begin to move the table closer to the kitchen table, bumping it a few feet in the right direction every meal. Once they are comfortable in the eating environment, they can transition to eating at the designated table.

Action Plan: Choose a location where you can consistently eat. Set a realistic goal for how many times you can eat meals here in the next week.

How Often Kids Should Be Eating

Instituting a schedule for meals and snacks may not have been on your radar when you set out to improve your child's eating. It should have been! Boundaries around when your child eats increases the likelihood that they will try new food, helps them eat larger quantities and improves their behavior at meals.

Schedules aren't only about when eating happens, but also when it doesn't happen. Kids who eat on demand throughout the day are perpetually in a state of hunger limbo. Snackers will eat just enough to cap their appetites. When a full meal comes around, they tend to not be hungry enough. Because children are born with an innate ability to adhere to their hunger cues, they have no motivation or reason to eat simply because it is mealtime. Frequent snackers might seem picky just because they're not hungry enough to be interested in trying table food.

Incessant grazing also reinforces the idea that children can eat whenever and often whatever they want. They learn that they don't need to eat at a meal because they can snack whenever they want. Informal eating opportunities can be more appealing because kids tend to get access to highly preferred snack foods and they're not required to sit still for a long period of time to eat them.

Limiting intake between meals allows your child to become hungry and improves the chance that they will eat what you serve at meals. It also gives them the opportunity to practice eating the right portion sizes. Ultimately, the boundaries and consistency of an eating schedule provide the support children need to improve their diets and meet their nutritional needs.

Sticking to a schedule and limiting unplanned eating opportunities doesn't mean that all meals and snacks need to occur at exactly the same time every day. You always have flexibility. Aim to space the start of meals and snacks two and a half to three hours apart.

Your child might ask for food between meals, especially if they are used to eating on demand. I recommend serving only water between scheduled meals and snacks. If they ask for food between meals, share the time of the next meal. Older kids might like to see a timer or know the exact time of the meal. Younger kids can use a verbal warning. Every child is different, so use your best judgment to assess if they're eating enough. You are in charge of the schedule and you might need to adjust the timing and frequency of mealtimes.

Action Plan: Begin to map out a schedule for your family's meals and snacks. Establishing exact times is less important than adhering to a general guideline. Remember, you'll likely be spacing the start of meals two and a half to three hours apart.

Shared Meals

Eat with your child as often as possible. The more you do, the more benefits you'll see. Family meals are linked to tons of benefits. Most important to your current agenda, children are more likely to try foods that they've seen their family or peers enjoy, and children who eat with their family regularly have better nutritional intake and tend to consume larger quantities of fruits and vegetables.

Aim to share at least one meal per day. This will provide your selective eater with exposure to new foods and regular opportunities to observe healthy eating habits. Plus, the strategies to encourage your child to try new foods that you'll be putting into play later are more effective if you're eating together.

It does not matter whether your mealtime guest list varies or whether a family meal contains only two people. It's also completely fine if your shared meal is not dinner. It's the experience that counts, not the details.

Action Plan: Choose a meal you can share with your child. Set a realistic goal for how many times you can eat together in the next week.

How to Serve Meals and What to Serve

Select one menu for the entire family. Serve the same foods for everyone. Preferably, do this at all meals, but definitely at the main meal that you are sharing together. When the family shares one menu, even one that contains specific dishes for individual eaters, it conveys the message that your child can eat anything.

Always include at least one food your child will eat with every meal, even if it's just a side dish. Meals should include a variety of foods, typically a protein, a carbohydrate (starch) and a vegetable and/or fruit. Be sure to include a variety of colors and textures.

I recommend serving meals family style. Instead of pre-plating each individual's meal, bring all of the food to the table in serving dishes like at a buffet, which allows each eater to serve themself. The act of serving oneself necessitates an interaction. Even if a child is just passing a dish, they'll still be bringing the food close to their bodies, will likely be looking at it and might even end up smelling it. Over time, these interactions can increase a child's willingness to eat a novel food. Serving also reinforces the eater's control over what and how much they might eat. If serving is too advanced for your child, ask them to guide the portion you put on their plate.

When meal planning, set a goal to incorporate daily variety for preferred and new foods. Many extreme picky eaters tend to eat the same few foods on repeat. Seeing the same food prepared the exact same way day after day fuels a desire for control over food and reinforces a picky eating mentality. My rule is to avoid serving the same food two days in a row (or three days in a row if your child eats a larger selection of foods). The exception is fruits and vegetables.

If your child's diet is too narrow to accomplish this now, keep it in mind as you move forward. Page 196 also has suggestions for altering the presentation of preferred foods.

Action Plan: Consider meals your family typically eats and what your picky eater typically eats. Make a plan for serving meals that incorporate both groups of food.

Appropriate Portion Sizes

We tend to overestimate the amount of food that children need to eat. A child's stomach is only the size of their fist, so they really can't eat that much at one time. In general, kids require about one teaspoon of food from each food group (protein, carbohydrate and fruit/vegetable) for each year of their age at every meal. For example, if your child is four, they need four teaspoons from each food group for a total of 12 teaspoons of food at each meal (see page 83 for more details). That's a guideline, not a rule. If your child is consistently eating more or less than this amount, it is not an indication that something is wrong.

I always recommend starting off with small portion sizes. You can always provide seconds. Offering children large portions sets you both up for failure and disappoint-ment. Additionally, large portions, especially of new foods, can overwhelm skeptical eaters, further deterring them from eating.

Action Plan: Allow your child to serve themselves. You can guide their portions so they don't end up with too much and remind them that they can get more if they are still hungry. This will help them learn what portion is right for their body. If you are plating a meal, keep the teaspoon guide in mind and avoid crowding their plate.

Troubleshooting and Tips for Success

Check the Chair: Eating involves the entire body. The shoulders, trunk and lower body all play a role in your child's eating. It can be difficult for kids to chew and swallow appropriately when these areas are not supported. Eating at a table in a comfortable and supportive chair can help a child eat safely, focus on the food and enjoy the meal. The ideal setup creates 90-degree angles at your child's hips, knees and ankles.

What to Do If They Don't Eat: Remember that it is up to your child to decide how much and whether they eat. Give your child a warning when a meal is ending and reinforce that when the meal is done, regardless of how much they ate, the kitchen is closed until the next eating opportunity. Resist the urge to provide food outside of your planned schedule as this can devalue mealtimes and send the message that your child can dictate the *when, what* and *where* of eating.

If your child eats inadequately during a meal and you are concerned, or as you are transitioning to the DOR and scheduled mealtimes, you might want to offer additional snacks. Just be careful to avoid making it seem like it's a result of them skipping the meal.

If you notice your child is refusing to eat for a period of time, is losing weight or is impacted significantly in their day-to-day life, I suggest checking in with your doctor or a registered dietitian.

Your Role in Mealtimes: In addition to managing the *what, when* and *where* of feeding, you are serving as a role model for your child during mealtimes. It is your job not only to model the eating behavior you want to see but also to make eating easier for your child by keeping meals positive, fun and free of pressure. I know that mealtimes with a particular eater can feel anything but calm. Although it's easier said than done, put any negative thoughts about what or how much your child is eating aside.

Not only does everyone have more fun when meals are pleasant, but it might also improve your child's eating.

Stress and anxiety can negatively impact appetite. I suggest avoiding the following behaviors to foster a positive and comfortable meal environment:

- Responding positively or negatively to how your child is eating. Instead, remain neutral and ignore any mealtime behaviors that you don't want to see repeated.
- Expressing judgment about your child's behavior or how they are eating.
- Discussing your child's eating habits or how much they eat during the meal.

Managing Sensory Stressors at Mealtimes

If your child's eating difficulties have a sensory component, it's possible that things that have nothing to do with food interfere with their ability to sit comfortably at meals. Look to triggers like sounds, lighting and smells that may be present during meals. You might never have noticed them, but they're all over. If your child is sensitive to any of these factors, consider some of the following adjustments to make the experience more comfortable for them.

If your child is sensitive to smells:

- Suggest they avoid the kitchen while food is cooking.
- Avoid cooking with strong spices and aromatics (onion, garlic, curry).
- Prepare food ahead of mealtimes.
- Serve cold or warm dishes (heat intensifies smell).
- Cover serving dishes.
- Keep serving plates away from your child's seat.

If your child is sensitive to noise:

- Play soothing music at meals.
- Seat them next to a quiet chewer.
- Use softer utensils and plates, such as bamboo, instead of metal or ceramic.

- Provide sound-muffling headphones for meals.
- Silence electronics, including phones, during the meal.
- Turn off timers or auditory disruptions that may go off during the meal.

If your child is sensitive to touch:
- Provide preferred utensils.
- Make sure they are comfortable with the material of the chair.
- Experiment with different food preparations so they can avoid touching ones that bother them.
- Keep a napkin nearby to wipe unwanted foods away.

If your child is sensitive to visual disruptions or has trouble with attention:
- Be sure to eat in a consistent location that is reserved for eating.
- Cover serving dishes.
- Serve food in opaque dishes.
- Position your child's back to any visible distractions.
- Clear the table and surrounding space of anything unrelated to the meal.
- Keep the mealtime routine and setup consistent.
- Cover blinking lights that may be coming from the kitchen or other nearby electronics.
- Turn off the TV.
- Dim the lights.

Selecting and Serving New Foods

Adding new foods occurs on two levels. One is passive—foods that are naturally included in your family meal. The other is active—introducing your child to specific foods that are not already a mealtime staple. I'm sure you can think of dozens of foods you'd love for your child to eat.

When you're seeking to expand a child's restricted diet, though, it's best to be intentional about the first foods that you introduce. I suggest selecting one of the following areas to focus on:

Foods that fill a nutritional gap. For example, high-calorie foods if your child is underweight.

Foods that will make your life easier. For example, ones that are easy to prepare or that your child can pack for lunch.

Foods that your family regularly eats. This is a helpful focus if your goal is to stop preparing multiple meals.

Foods your child used to eat. Previously preferred foods tend to be easier to reintroduce and are a more reliable way to quickly incorporate new foods into your child's diet.

Within these parameters, I suggest thinking about foods your child will be most likely to eat. For more details, refer to page 101 (Building Food Bridges).

CHAPTER 9

Strategies for Introducing New Food to the Most Extreme Picky Eaters

Include a New Food at Every Meal

Aim to serve a new food at every meal and snack. During your shared meals, this is any nonpreferred food. During meals that your child is eating alone, I recommend only serving one new food that you've selected using the previously described strategies as well as the ones below. Remember that the more your child is exposed to new foods, the more likely they will be to eat them.

Make Small Changes to Preferred Foods

In addition to rotating the daily menu as much as possible, I recommend making small changes to the foods that your child is regularly eating. These variations will promote a flexible mindset and help break down rigidity that might be holding your child back from eating at restaurants or enjoying different brands of preferred foods. It's another strategy to build a bridge from preferred foods to novel ones.

The more severe your child's eating difficulties are, the smaller these changes will need to be. Aim for the most significant change that your child can tolerate. Think about introducing different brands, colors, flavors, textures, sizes or presentations. Making small adjustments to these areas is a good place to start.

Remember to still include at least one preferred food in its preferred form. For the best chances of success, you might want to try offering choices (i.e., Would you prefer your sandwich cut into squares or triangles?) and serving the changed and unchanged versions of the food together. If it's not going well, you might be offering too significant of a change or changing the food too frequently. Try scaling back in either area.

Start Small

When introducing new foods, smaller is always better. Think about not only the portion size but also the size of the piece that you're offering. The idea is to start small and gradually increase the portion or bite size as your child gains comfort with the novel food.

Think first about providing a very small individual piece of a new food. When I say small, I mean really small. For the most extreme picky eaters, I might start with a food cut as small as a grain of rice or a pea. Once they are tolerating this teeny portion, you can gradually increase the bite size. When your child is eating a typical bite, increase the total portion until they are able to eat an age-appropriate serving.

Mix and Fade

I'm frequently asked how to encourage a child with rigid texture preferences to welcome new foods outside of their comfortable texture. My answer? Start small. I'm all about incremental changes when it comes to introducing new foods. You'll notice this in most of my recommendations. Small changes are not only easier for extreme picky eaters to manage, but they also promote the natural development of a new preference by slowly acclimating a child to a new eating experience. It is an ideal strategy for children who experience neophobia, strong sensory aversions, eating anxiety and negative reactions when encountering a new food. Be sure to keep the changes gradual and to only introduce a change once your child has willingly accepted a new food at least three consecutive times. A few examples are:

Chocolate milk to plain: Add plain milk to chocolate in a ratio of 1:10. Progressively increase the amount of plain milk until your child accepts it on its own.

Raw carrots to cooked: Beginning with a raw carrot in its preferred form, gradually increase the cooking time so you are serving carrots that are more and more tender over time.

Beef to turkey meatballs: Incorporate turkey into the mix so it is just barely detectable. Continue to add more each time you make them until the meatball is 100 percent turkey.

Plain pizza to pizza with toppings: Offer the usual pizza with one tiny topping piece. Continue to increase the presence of toppings and their bite size until a child is accepting pizza with toppings.

Pairing New and Preferred Foods

New foods are better received when presented with preferred foods. Offer a novel food alongside a preferred food, or combine the new with the preferred food (like in the pizza example above) so the preferred food becomes a vehicle for the new. The combination of new and preferred makes the new food more approachable, and the preferred food can mask the texture and taste of the nonpreferred food. Remember, this is just a transitional bridge to facilitate tasting. The goal is to ultimately phase out the preferred food.

If your child likes dips, this is a great time to use them.

Find dip suggestions and ideas for using dips effectively on page 180.

Be transparent if you are using a preferred food vehicle. I do not recommend hiding a new food in a preferred food (i.e., pureeing vegetables in a favorite sauce) without telling your child. The intention of using a preferred food vehicle is to decrease your child's discomfort and train their taste buds so they can eventually eat the novel food on its own.

As with the above strategies, you might need to start small with an almost unnoticeable portion of new food.

A Parent's New Food Tracker

Consider tracking your progress as you introduce new foods. Tracking keeps you sane. It allows you to see what you're doing, how many times you've tried something and how each food introduction went. Additionally, tracking allows you to visualize your progress, which will feel so good and encourage you to keep working. Some parents like to keep their tracker on their phone and others prefer to have a hard copy. Whichever way you prefer, consider including the following information:

- Date
- Meal
- Food
- Food preparation
- Size offered
- Child's response
- Child's interaction
- Food eaten? Yes/No
- Quantity eaten
- Number of exposures

CHAPTER 10

Encouraging Kids to Eat and Interact with New Foods

New food exposures and fun, hands-on experiences with new foods will acclimate your child's sensory system and, over time, inspire your child to eat. The following sensory experiences and fun interactions with novel foods are ideas to inspire you. I don't intend them as prescriptions to be followed precisely. Pick and choose what is fun and feasible for your family, or create your own plan.

These activities can be extremely effective; however, they work best when used in conjunction with the more targeted approaches and mealtime foundation discussed in Chapter 7.

In addition to the activities listed on the following pages, cooking is one of my favorite techniques for encouraging interactions with novel foods. You can find more details on page 210.

"Can" Phrases

When introducing new foods, I recommend avoiding pressure. That gets tricky when you're trying to encourage your child to engage with something new. Try replacing requests and demands with "can" phrases. These suggestions empower a child and reveal opportunities that can increase their comfort with foods while they're working up to eating them. There's no limit to how or when you use these phrases. Some suggestions include:

You can . . .
- describe what it looks like.
- poke it with a fork.
- pass it to me.
- move it off your plate.
- smell it.
- see how it feels with the tip of your finger.
- hold it in your hand to see how heavy it is.
- squish it between your fingers.
- lick it.
- take a bite if you're ready.
- spit it out.

Keep the Food Conversation Open

Many extreme picky eaters shy away from eating or engaging with new foods because they can't anticipate what the experience of doing so will be like. To help them make connections and learn what to expect, create a dialogue about food. Outside of mealtimes, get to know new foods by comparing and contrasting different forms of the same food using all of the senses. Start by discussing the smell, feel and look of the foods. Then move on to tasting them if possible. Invite your child to assist with the different preparations to enhance the sensory experience. Some foods to use for this activity include:

1. A whole carrot with greens, peeled carrots, diced carrots, carrot rounds, carrot spears, crinkle-cut carrot "chips," shredded carrots, roasted carrots, steamed carrots, pureed carrots and carrot juice

2. Chicken nuggets, breaded chicken, chicken strips, grilled chicken, shredded chicken, chicken patties and chicken sausage

3. Frozen, fresh, freeze-dried and dried strawberries

4. Applesauce, apple chips, soft dried apple, whole apples, apple slices, apple wedges, peeled apples and baked apples

Additionally, talking about a food's taste, texture and smell, and even describing the process of eating and experiencing food with your senses, can help train a child's expectations. When doing this, be sure to deliver information in a neutral and casual way. Some examples:

- "The avocado is so creamy."
- "These radishes are crunchy like a chip, but they don't crumble in my mouth."
- "I am using my front teeth to bite off a tiny piece of this tart apple. It's crunchy and the inside is wet."
- "The bread on my grilled cheese is a little crisp, but the cheese is soft and warm. It stretches when I take a bite."
- "This yogurt is tart and smooth."
- "This peach is so juicy I have to slurp when I'm eating it."
- "This cracker is very easy to chew because it dissolves in my mouth."
- "I'm chewing the sandwich until it's soft before I swallow it."
- "This cucumber is watery like melon."

Hands-On Food Play

Playing will help your child understand and feel more comfortable with food. The goal is to use play to encourage your child to start engaging with food. Keep in mind a child's typical ladder to acceptance, which will help you understand how to help them move closer to eating.

Aversion and avoidance

- May not tolerate a food on their plate, at the table, in the room or even in the house
- Upset when the food comes too close or across their "boundary" lines
- Might gag or throw up at the sight or smell of food

Tolerance

- Will tolerate food on the table or their plate (with certain conditions)
- Might ignore the food, but is okay knowing it is around

Engagement

- Looks at food
- Shows some interest
- Pokes at food with a utensil
- Can discuss properties (color, texture, size, shape)
- No direct touching

Exploration

- Touches with a body part (fingertip) in some way
- Interacts with, such as pulls apart or crushes
- Feels and explores with curiosity and play
- Smells
- Touches part of their face with the food
- Kisses
- Within this, the closer the exploration is to the face and head, the further along they are in the process

Tasting

- May hold in lips, teeth, mouth
- May chew and spit out

Eating

- Eats the food (even only one or two bites)

Your job is to identify your child's current stage of acceptance with a new food. You can't suggest they lick something if they're not even looking at it yet. So, begin at their stage of acceptance and model how to engage with food in a playful manner to gently push them up the ladder of acceptance. Just pretend you're playing with toys. The more you practice, the easier this will become.

This technique tends to work best for kids under the age of seven. You can incorporate food play during a meal when you notice your child ignoring or stagnating with a particular food. You can also dedicate time outside of meals. Extremely hesitant eaters might prefer to play outside of mealtimes when they will feel less expectation for them to eat.

Find ideas to inspire your food play on page 129.

Food Play Outside of Mealtimes

What you need:

- 1 plate for each participant (including the grown-up)
- 3 to 10 foods, including at least one preferred food, enough for each participant
- Napkins available for each participant
- Tools (i.e., cookie cutters, cups, food picks, etc.)

How to:

1. Prepare the foods beforehand and set them on plates. Each plate will have a portion of each food. Keep the plate out of the child's eyesight and reach, if possible.

2. Tell them it's playtime with food. Stress that you're not eating, just playing.

3. Starting with a preferred food, present one food at a time for each participant.

4. Begin playing with or exploring the food and invite your child to participate. Follow their lead and work through the ladder of acceptance.

5. Watch your child's reactions. When your child reaches

their limit with a food, introduce the next food. You can incorporate that food into the same play scheme or create a new one.

6. Stop playing when your child loses interest or seems to have reached their capacity. It's better to end on a good note than to push them past their limit.

Food Play During Mealtimes
What you need:
- The mealtime foods
- Napkins available for each participant

How to:
1. Designate time to incorporate play into your regular meal routine or spontaneously play when your child is not initiating engagement with a food.

2. Starting at their level of acceptance, begin playing or exploring the food, encouraging them to advance up their ladder of acceptance.

3. Stop when your child loses interest, eats the food or it is time to move on with the meal.

Embrace the Mess!
It's okay to get messy. The whole concept behind food play is getting your hands dirty. Mess is inevitable and it's actually a good sign. Resist your urge to keep things tidy and try to avoid putting boundaries on the type of play due to concerns about mess. If it's a big deal, play on a mat, place mat or leakproof tablecloth.

Tips for Success with Food Play
- Get silly.
- Tap into your child's interests.
- Avoid asking them to do something. Instead, model or use "can" phrases.
- Always participate alongside your child.

- Follow their lead. If your child skips phases, jump ahead with them. If you see signs that they're ready to be done, wrap up the activity.
- If they're not joining in, take a step down the ladder to make the task easier for them or try a new angle.

Food Explorers

This is a take on food play for ages seven and up. While older kids still benefit immensely from hands-on exposure with food, not all will enjoy entering into the realm of make-believe. Putting a scientific spin on their activity not only encourages them to interact with food, but it also helps them learn about food and overcome mental blocks to eating.

Mealtime food exploring uses objective examination to guide new interactions with food. As an explorer, it is important to approach food with an open mind and use objective, scientific language to describe findings.

You can examine and then describe food using objective language or conduct mini experiments to move up the ladder of acceptance.

Strive to make mealtime food exploring come about organically. Notice how your child is engaging with a food and consider ways to get them to intensify their interaction. Like food play, this activity can also be conducted outside of meals.

The duration of food exploring is less important than the frequency.

What you need (outside of mealtimes):

- 1 to 5 foods, including at least one preferred food, for each participant
- Any tools that you may want to use for your experiments

How to:

1. Start with your child's preferred food. Either pose a question to guide your exploration along the ladder of

acceptance or use your child's stage on the ladder to create a simple experiment. See suggestions below.

2. Once you've finished with the preferred food, move on to novel foods. You'll know your child is done when they're either eating the food or are no longer comfortable progressing up the ladder.

Some ideas:
- Describe the food's physical appearance (color, shape, etc.), texture, weight, smell and/or taste.

Explore comparisons:
- Which do you think is softer?
- Let's see which is heaviest.

Hypothesize:
- I wonder whether the sweet potato will taste sweet.
- Rate the intensity of sensory discoveries as big, medium or small.
- How many times do you think you'd have to chew the bread until it's soft?
- How hard do you think you have to push to cut the broccoli?

Experiment:
- Will the meat loaf taste different cut into thick or thin slices?
- How will adding ketchup change the flavor?
- If we drizzle gravy on the turkey, does the texture change?

Growing a Vegetable Garden
While teaching nutrition in New York City public schools, I learned the key to getting the most vegetable-resistant kids to talk about, touch and even eat vegetables. The secret? It's planting a garden.

Kids are excited, proud and curious about foods they help grow. Additionally, research shows that planting a food garden improves a child's diet, sensory development

and education. Children who garden show advancements in three major areas: knowledge about fruits and
vegetables, willingness to try fruits and vegetables and
preference for the fruits and vegetables they grow.[79]
For such a simple activity, those are pretty significant
results.

Like so many things, gardening sounds daunting, but it
doesn't require as much space, time, effort, skill or financial
investment as we often think. Think of "gardening" as
growing just one thing that you can eat. And then get
started with these six easy steps:

1. Discuss where you will start your garden. Do you have
beds or will you use pots?

2. What will you grow? I look for two things when selecting
seeds: Are they easy to grow and will they fit with your
space and climate? It helps to choose things that are
not fussy about the soil or climate, are low-maintenance
and don't require starting indoors. Carrots, radishes, green
beans and lettuces are very simple. Some veggies like
beets require deep soil, and others like zucchini develop
long vines that take up a lot of space aboveground, so
take all of these factors into consideration.

3. Make a list of all of the materials you will need for your
garden and head to the store. Your child can be in charge
of checking items off the list.

4. Set aside a time to plant your garden.

5. Make a plan for maintaining your garden. Address how
often plants will need to be watered and how long they
need to grow.

6. Monitor your plants' growth with your child and help
them track the progress. You might remind them that
it takes time for plants to grow (just as it takes time to
learn to like new foods!).

Children love watching their seeds grow. If your child is engaged with the growing process, capitalize on their excitement and use the opportunity to teach them about nutrition while also expanding their palate. During the growing process, you can note how plants require sun, soil and water to grow big and strong. Point out that your child needs nutrients from tasty and nutritious foods like the one you're growing to grow big and strong.

When the vegetables are grown, have your child do as much of the harvesting as possible. See if they want to sample their harvest straight from the garden. Encourage sensory exploration: Describe the food's color, texture, weight and smell. Finally, plan a meal or snack around your harvest. It's a bonus if your child helps prepare it.

Food Art

Making art with food engages a child's senses and sparks positive connections. When being creative, they're bound to get dirty and engage with food in a way they might not if they met it on their plate at mealtime. Try some of these ideas:

- Make your own potato head.
- Create stamps from hardy fruits and vegetables like potatoes, carrots, beets and apples; use these on paper or on the body. You can use ink or other food as paint. Beets create their own stamps when they're wet.
- Create a picture by gluing dry foods like pasta, dried beans, crackers, nuts, freeze-dried veggies and dried fruit on paper.
- Make necklaces of popcorn and fresh or dried fruits and vegetables.
- Create a food rainbow.
- Paint using sauces, condiments, dressings or purees. Use sturdy or textured foods like carrot sticks, pretzels, celery or broccoli as paintbrushes.

- Create bite art using foods like apples, soft bread, cheese, cucumbers and bell peppers, which retain their shape when bitten into. Use different teeth and varying amounts of pressure to see the different patterns you can create.

A Personal Kid's Tasting Tracker

Recording their progress can be a huge motivator for some kids. You can create a food tracker for them or have them make their own. Use different colors, stickers or drawings to record each taste.

One word of warning if using a tracker: Be careful not to use the tracker as a bargaining piece. It can be a fun extra but should not be used to coerce your child into eating.

What you need:
- Piece of paper
- Markers
- Stickers to record progress (optional)

How to:
1. Create a grid with at least 11 columns and as many rows as will fit on the paper.

2. Using the leftmost column, record new foods your child is learning to like.

3. Each time your child completes the goal task (i.e., eating, tasting or interacting with a new food), they can add a mark to the column next to that food.

Endnotes

[1] De Cosmi, V., S. Scaglioni, and C. Agostoni. "Early taste experiences and later food choices." *Nutrients* 9.2 (2017): 107.

[2] Harris, G. "Development of taste and food preferences in children." *Current Opinion in Clinical Nutrition & Metabolic Care* 11.3 (2008): 315–319.

[3] Coulthard, H., and D. Thakker. "Enjoyment of tactile play is associated with lower food neophobia in preschool children." *Journal of the Academy of Nutrition and Dietetics* 115.7 (2015): 1134–1140.

[4] The National Center on Addiction and Substance Abuse at Columbia University. "The importance of family dinners VIII." September 2012. Accessed March 16, 2020. https://www.centeronaddiction.org/addiction-research/reports/importance-of-family-dinners-2012.

[5] Harper, L. V., and K. M. Sanders. "The effect of adults' eating on young children's acceptance of unfamiliar foods." *Journal of Experimental Child Psychology* 20.2 (1975): 206–214.

[6] Hobden, K., and P. Pliner. "Effects of a model on food neophobia in humans." *Appetite* 25.2 (1995): 101–114.

[7] Brown, R., and J. Ogden. "Children's eating attitudes and behaviour: A study of the modelling and control theories of parental influence." *Health Education Research* 19.3 (2004): 261–271.

[8] Taylor, C. M., et al. "Picky/fussy eating in children: Review of definitions, assessment, prevalence and dietary intakes." *Appetite* 95 (2015): 349–359.

[9] Reau, N. R., et al. "Infant and toddler feeding patterns and problems: Normative data and a new direction." *Journal of Developmental and Behavioral Pediatrics* 17.3 (1996): 149–153.

[10] Reed, D. R., and A. Knaapila. "Genetics of taste and smell: Poisons and pleasures." *Progress in Molecular Biology and Translational Science* 94 (2010): 213–240.

[11] Needleman, R. "Growth and development." In *Nelson Textbook of Pediatrics*. 16th ed. Edited by R. E. Behrman, R. M. Kliegman, and H. B. Jensen, 23–50. Philadelphia: W. B. Saunders, 2000.

[12] Walton, K., et al. "Time to re-think picky eating?: A relational approach to understanding picky eating." *International Journal of Behavioral Nutrition and Physical Activity* 14.1 (2017): 62.

13   Toomey, K., and E. Ross. "When children won't eat: Picky eaters vs. problem feeders." Conference, Philadelphia, May 14–17, 2019.

14   Birch, L. L., and D. W. Marlin. "I don't like it; I never tried it: Effects of exposure on two-year-old children's food preferences." *Appetite* 3.4 (1982): 353–360.

15   Dunbar, R. I. M. "Breaking bread: The functions of social eating." *Adaptive Human Behavior and Physiology* 3.3 (2017): 198–211.

16   Toomey, K. A., and E. S. Ross. "SOS approach to feeding." *Perspectives on Swallowing and Swallowing Disorders (Dysphagia)* 20.3 (2011): 82–87.

17   Barthomeuf, L., S. Droit-Volet, and S. Rousset. "How emotions expressed by adults' faces affect the desire to eat liked and disliked foods in children compared to adults." *British Journal of Developmental Psychology* 30.2 (2012): 253–266.

18   Dunn, W. "The impact of sensory processing abilities on the daily lives of young children and their families: A conceptual model." *Infants & Young Children* 9 (1997): 23–35.

19   Smith, A. M., et al. "Food choices of tactile defensive children." *Nutrition* 21.1 (2005): 14–19.

20   Coulthard, H., and J. Blissett. "Fruit and vegetable consumption in children and their mothers: Moderating effects of child sensory sensitivity." *Appetite* 52.2 (2009): 410–415.

21   Farrow, C. V., and H. Coulthard. "Relationships between sensory sensitivity, anxiety and selective eating in children." *Appetite* 58.3 (2012): 842–846.

22   Smith, A. M., et al. "Food choices of tactile defensive children." *Nutrition* 21.1 (2005): 14–19.

23   Ben-Sasson, A., et al. "A meta-analysis of sensory modulation symptoms in individuals with autism spectrum disorders." *Journal of Autism and Developmental Disorders* 39.1 (2009): 1–11.

24   Ahn, R. R., et al. "Prevalence of parents' perceptions of sensory processing disorders among kindergarten children." *American Journal of Occupational Therapy* 58.3 (2004): 287–293.

25   Kähkönen, K., et al. "Sensory-based food education in early childhood education and care, willingness to choose and eat fruit and vegetables, and the moderating role of maternal education and food neophobia." *Public Health Nutrition* 21.13 (2018): 2443–2453.

26   Nederkoorn, C., A. Jansen, and R. C. Havermans. "Feel your food: The influence of tactile sensitivity on picky eating in children." *Appetite* 84 (2015): 7–10.

27   Eldeghaidy, S., et al. "An automated method to detect and quantify fungiform papillae in the human tongue: Validation and relationship to

phenotypical differences in taste perception." *Physiology & Behavior* 184 (2018): 226–234.

[28] Bell, K. I., and B. J. Tepper. "Short-term vegetable intake by young children classified by 6-n-propylthoiuracil bitter-taste phenotype." *The American Journal of Clinical Nutrition* 84.1 (2006): 245–251.

[29] Meyerhof, W., et al. "Human bitter taste perception." *Chemical Senses* 30, suppl 1 (2005): i14–i15.

[30] Mennella, J. A., M. Y. Pepino, and D. R. Reed. "Genetic and environmental determinants of bitter perception and sweet preferences." *Pediatrics* 115.2 (2005): e216–e222.

[31] Drewnowski, A., and C. Gomez-Carneros. "Bitter taste, phytonutrients, and the consumer: A review." *The American Journal of Clinical Nutrition* 72.6 (2000): 1424–1435.

[32] Koivisto, U. K., and P. O. Sjödén. "Reasons for rejection of food items in Swedish families with children aged 2–17." *Appetite* 26.1 (1996): 89–104.

[33] Carruth, B. R., et al. "Prevalence of picky eaters among infants and toddlers and their caregivers' decisions about offering a new food." *Journal of the American Dietetic Association* 104 , suppl 1 (2004): 57–64.

[34] Mallan, K. M., et al. "Feeding a fussy eater: Examining longitudinal bidirectional relationships between child fussy eating and maternal feeding practices." *Journal of Pediatric Psychology* 43.10 (2018): 1138–1146.

[35] Kleinman, R. E., ed. *Pediatric Nutrition Handbook*. 6th ed. Elk Grove Village, IL: American Academy of Pediatrics, 2009.

[36] Sebastian, R. S., L. E. Cleveland, and J. D. Goldman. "Effect of snacking frequency on adolescents' dietary intakes and meeting national recommendations." *Journal of Adolescent Health* 42.5 (2008): 503–511.

[37] Larson-Nath, C. M., and P. S. Goday. "Failure to thrive: A prospective study in a pediatric gastroenterology clinic." *Journal of Pediatric Gastroenterology and Nutrition* 62.6 (2016): 907–913.

[38] Galloway, A. T., et al. "'Finish your soup': Counterproductive effects of pressuring children to eat on intake and affect." *Appetite* 46.3 (2006): 318–323.

[39] Carruth, B. R., et al. "Prevalence of picky eaters among infants and toddlers and their caregivers' decisions about offering a new food." *Journal of the American Dietetic Association* 104 , suppl 1 (2004): 57–64.

[40] Cornish, E. "A balanced approach towards healthy eating in autism." *Journal of Human Nutrition and Dietetics* 11.6 (1998): 501–509.

[41] Ellis, J. M., et al. "Recollections of pressure to eat during childhood, but not picky eating, predict young adult eating behavior." *Appetite* 97 (2016): 58–63.

42   Coon, K. A., et al. "Relationships between use of television during meals and children's food consumption patterns." *Pediatrics* 107.1 (2001): e7.

43   Powell, F., et al. "The importance of mealtime structure for reducing child food fussiness." *Maternal & Child Nutrition* 13.2 (2017): e12296.

44   Anzman-Frasca, S., et al. "Repeated exposure and associative conditioning promote preschool children's liking of vegetables." *Appetite* 58.2 (2012): 543–553.

45   Fisher, J. O., et al. "Offering 'dip' promotes intake of a moderately liked raw vegetable among preschoolers with genetic sensitivity to bitterness." *Journal of the Academy of Nutrition and Dietetics* 112.2 (2012): 235–245.

46   Pliner, P., and C. Stallberg-White. "'Pass the ketchup, please': Familiar flavors increase children's willingness to taste novel foods." *Appetite* 34.1 (2000): 95–103.

47   Loewen, R., and P. Pliner. "Effects of prior exposure to palatable and unpalatable novel foods on children's willingness to taste other novel foods." *Appetite* 32.3 (1999): 351–366.

48   Toomey, K. "Steps to Eating." Handout presented at "When children won't eat: Picky eaters vs. problem feeders." Conference, Philadelphia, May 14–17, 2019.

49   Smith, A. M., et al. "Food choices of tactile defensive children." *Nutrition* 21.1 (2005): 14–19.

50   Leekam, S. R., et al. "Describing the sensory abnormalities of children and adults with autism." *Journal of Autism and Developmental Disorders* 37.5 (2007): 894–910.

51   Miller, L. J., D. A. Fuller, and J. Roetenberg. *Sensational Kids: Hope and Help for Children with Sensory Processing Disorder (SPD)*. New York: Penguin, 2014.

52   Fishbein, M., et al. "Food chaining: A systematic approach for the treatment of children with feeding aversion." *Nutrition in Clinical Practice* 21.2 (2006): 182–184.

53   Cunningham-Sabo, L., and B. Lohse. "Impact of a school-based cooking curriculum for fourth-grade students on attitudes and behaviors is influenced by gender and prior cooking experience." *Journal of Nutrition Education and Behavior* 46.2 (2014): 110–120.

54   Van der Horst, K., A. Ferrage, and A. Rytz. "Involving children in meal preparation: Effects on food intake." *Appetite* 79 (2014): 18–24.

55   Cullen, K. W., et al. "Achieving fruit, juice, and vegetable recipe preparation goals influences consumption by 4th grade students." *International Journal of Behavioral Nutrition and Physical Activity* 4.1 (2007): 28.

56   Hermann, J. R., et al. "After-school gardening improves children's reported vegetable intake and physical activity." *Journal of Nutrition Education and Behavior* 38.3 (2006): 201–202.

57   Van der Horst, K. "Overcoming picky eating: Eating enjoyment as a central aspect of children's eating behaviors." *Appetite* 58.2 (2012): 567–574.

58   Satter, E. *Child of Mine: Feeding with Love and Good Sense.* Boulder, CO: Bull Publishing Company, 2012.

59   Berge, J. M., et al. "Structural and interpersonal characteristics of family meals: Associations with adolescent body mass index and dietary patterns." *Journal of the Academy of Nutrition and Dietetics* 113.6 (2013): 816–822.

60   Piernas, C., and B. M. Popkin. "Trends in snacking among US children." *Health Affairs* 29.3 (2010): 398–404.

61   Finnane, J. M., et al. "Mealtime structure and responsive feeding practices are associated with less food fussiness and more food enjoyment in children." *Journal of Nutrition Education and Behavior* 49.1 (2017): 11–18.

62   Hammons, A. J., and B. H. Fiese. "Is frequency of shared family meals related to the nutritional health of children and adolescents?" *Pediatrics* 127.6 (2011): e1565–e1574.

63   The National Center on Addiction and Substance Abuse at Columbia University. "The importance of family dinners VIII." September 2012. Accessed March 16, 2020. https://www.centeronaddiction.org/addiction-research/reports/importance-of-family-dinners-2012.

64   Kähkönen, K., et al. "Sensory-based food education in early childhood education and care, willingness to choose and eat fruit and vegetables, and the moderating role of maternal education and food neophobia." *Public Health Nutrition* 21.13 (2018): 2443–2453.

65   Skinner, J. D., et al. "Mealtime communication patterns of infants from 2 to 24 months of age." *Journal of Nutrition Education* 30.1 (1998): 8–16.

66   Satter, E. *Child of Mine: Feeding with Love and Good Sense.* Boulder, CO: Bull Publishing Company, 2012.

67   Snow, C. E., and D. E. Beals. "Mealtime talk that supports literacy development." *New Directions for Child and Adolescent Development* 111 (2006): 51–66.

68   Story, M., and D. Neumark-Sztainer. "A perspective on family meals: Do they matter?" *Nutrition Today* 40.6 (2005): 261–266.

69   Owen, J. P., et al. "Abnormal white matter microstructure in children with sensory processing disorders." *Neuroimage: Clinical* 2 (2013): 844–853.

70   Mascola, A. J., S. W. Bryson, and W. S. Agras. "Picky eating during childhood: A longitudinal study to age 11 years." *Eating Behaviors* 11.4 (2010): 253-257.

71   Carruth, B. R., and J. D. Skinner. "Revisiting the picky eater phenomenon: Neophobic behaviors of young children." *Journal of the American College of Nutrition* 19.6 (2000): 771-780.

72   Jacobi, C., et al. "Behavioral validation, precursors, and concomitants of picky eating in childhood." *Journal of the American Academy of Child & Adolescent Psychiatry* 42.1 (2003): 76-84.

73   Esparo, G., et al. "Feeding problems in nursery children: Prevalence and psychosocial factors." *Acta Paediatrica* 93.5 (2004): 663-668.

74   Pescud, M., and S. Pettigrew. "Parents' experiences with hiding vegetables as a strategy for improving children's diets." *British Food Journal* 116.12 (2014): 1853-1863.

75   Caraher, M., et al. "When chefs adopt a school? An evaluation of a cooking intervention in English primary schools." *Appetite* 62 (2013): 50-59.

76   Heim, S., J. Stang, and M. Ireland. "A garden pilot project enhances fruit and vegetable consumption among children." *Journal of the American Dietetic Association* 109.7 (2009): 1220-1226.

77   Loso, J., et al. "Gardening experience is associated with increased fruit and vegetable intake among first-year college students: A cross-sectional examination." *Journal of the Academy of Nutrition and Dietetics* 118.2 (2018): 275-283.

78   Lally, P., et al. "How are habits formed: Modelling habit formation in the real world." *European Journal of Social Psychology* 40.6 (2010): 998-1009.

79   Davis, K. L., and L. S. Brann. "Examining the benefits and barriers of instructional gardening programs to increase fruit and vegetable intake among preschool-age children." *Journal of Environmental and Public Health* 2017 (2017): 1-7.

Acknowledgments

My heartfelt thanks:

To my editor, Sarah, and the team at Page Street Publishing for helping me create this important project and giving me the opportunity to fulfill a dream many years in the making. I am so grateful for your guidance and support.

To my husband, David, for everything that you do, including being so patient and taking such good care of me while I put our lives on hold to work on this. Thank you for rooting for me, for ensuring I always took a lunch break from writing and for assuming more than your share of dinner making and grocery shopping as I hunkered down to write.

To my family, for your endless support and encouragement.

To the families I work with, for welcoming me into your lives and homes, knowing that we're about to embark on a long and challenging journey; it is such a privilege. Working together and seeing your child progress from a skeptical eater to one who can enjoy a variety of foods is always the best part of my day.

About the Author

Jennifer Friedman, MS, RD, is a registered dietitian who specializes in extreme picky eating. Jennifer received her bachelor of arts degree from McGill University and her master of science degree in nutrition from Columbia University Teachers College.

Known for her playful and approachable style, Jennifer has become a leading resource for parents and professionals working with children who struggle at mealtimes. She shares her insight on her website and blog, JennyFriedmanNutrition.com, and on social media @autism.nutritionist.

Index

A

activities
  bridges, building food, 101–103
  dips, 180–184
  food play, intentional, 129–132
  grocery games, 154–156
  tastes test, 47–48
allergies/restrictions, food, 157, 159, 166–167, 174, 179
appetite/hunger, 17, 24–25, 69–70, 135–137, 140–142, 150, 152–153, 162, 222
art, with food, 33, 244–245
attention
  looking for, 112–114
  paid to meals, 84–86, 193–195, 238
  span, 115, 165–166, 194, 228
autism/spectrum disorders, 8, 53, 77, 84, 92, 135, 185. See also special needs children

B

baked goods
  50, 79, 77, 106, 127, 148, 50, 77, 79, 106, 127, 148
brand selectivity, 79, 96–98, 149–150, 185–186, 203–204
breakfasts, 21–22, 26, 34, 62, 82, 144, 158, 161
bridges, food, 101–103

C

calories, 23–24, 69, 82–83, 141, 191, 229
"can" phrase, 235–236
chain, food, 101–103
Child of Mine (Satter), 162
cleanliness, 18–19, 93, 129, 170–171, 189
complementary feeding, 17
conversations, food, 235–237
cooking, 157, 186, 201–203, 210–213

D

desensitization. See sensory exploration
developmental stages, of eating. See feeding phases
dips, 33, 93, 137, 146, 176–177, 180–184

distractions, of eating environment 193–194, 142–143, 25–26, 81–86, 113, 193–194, 221
diversity, of food. See exposure to new foods
Division of Responsibility for Feeding, 9, 117, 136, 162, 219–221

E

environment, mealtime
  about, 68
  comfort of, 113–114
  distraction free (See distractions, of eating environment)
  locations of meals, 221 (See also location, of meals)
  safety of, 17, 114–115, 167, 225–226
  schedule of, 222–223, 226 (See also schedule, eating)
  sensory reactions to (See sensory processing impairments)
  shared meals and, 223–224 (See also family meals, shared)
  structure of, 142–144, 160–164
exploration, sensory. See sensory exploration
Exploring Plate, 121–123
exposure to new foods
  activities for, 92–93, 101–103, 139
  behavior changes and, 197–199
  diversity of, through family meals, 115–117
  fading and mixing, and, 232–233
  and food play, intentional, 92–94, 96–97
  and hunger, 144, 150
  intentional, 86–90
  levels of, 228–229, 232
  portions, shared from table, 169
  preferred food modifications, and, 95–96, 149–150, 231–232
  with preferred foods, 55, 62, 88–89, 96, 138–139, 175–176, 232–234
  reintroductions, 33, 95, 229
  side plates and, 196
  through sensory exploration, 144–147
  tips for, 216–217
  tracking, 234

F

fading out preferred foods
family meals, shared
    exposure, for additional
        opportunities for, 72,
        85, 115, 117, 119–120, 167,
        172–174, 231
    ideal, 223–224
    importance of, 22, 68, 70, 72, 143,
        223–224
    pressure-free, 161
    and sibling obstacles, 143
    social benefits of, 25, 27
    discomfort of, 205–207
feeding phases, 17, 90
feeding therapy. See Food Explorers
Fishbein, Mark, 9
flavors
    identification of, 17, 36–37, 47–48,
        55, 122, 146
    intensity, 30, 32, 59, 62–63, 178, 204
    sensitivity to, 52, 62–64, 227
Food Explorers, 26–34, 54–64, 68–69,
    241
Fraker, Cheri, 9

G

gag, 52, 185–186
gardens, 190, 201–202, 242–244
grocery shopping, 44, 144–145, 154–156,
    159

H

hands-on exploration. See sensory
    exploration
hunger/appetite. See appetite/hunger

I

illnesses, 19, 21
intake needs, 49–50, 58, 69–71, 83
introduction to new food. See exposure
    to new foods

J

junk food. See snacks

L

language, for food descriptions
    56-58, 135, 139, 241
limits, feeding and food, 23, 70
location, of meals, 25–26, 86, 106, 108–
    114, 142–143, 193–195, 221–222.
    See also school, eating at

M

meal prep, age-appropriate, 212–213
messes. See cleanliness
mixed food, 232–233
modeling eating behavior, 22–23, 26,
    85, 171, 226
multivitamins, 83–84, 191–192

N

noise, 210–211, 227–228. See also sound,
    of food
nutrition. See also calories; snacks
    development and, 24–25, 82–84,
        157–158, 229
    and dietary restrictions, 166–167
    increasing intake, 69, 71
    and roles, mealtime, 219–220
    snacking and, 135, 141, 222
    teaching, 229
    vitamins and, 192

O

oral sensitivities, 9, 20, 58

P

packaging, disguise of, 149
parents
    engagement of, 54–55, 110–111, 146,
        150, 161
    involvement in meal process, 108–
        109
    as models of eating behavior, 22–
        23, 26, 85, 226
    role of, 117, 187–188
phases, of picky eating, 24–25, 77–78
planning, meal, 118, 137–139, 144–145,
    224
plating, pre-, 120, 168, 224. See also
    serving meals
playing with food, intentional, as part
    of sensory exploration, 129–
    132, 237–241
portion sizes, 136, 225
preferred foods
    manipulation of, by parent, 151
    with meals, 117, 119, 169
    with new food introduction, 55,
        62, 88–89, 96, 138–139,
        175–176, 232–234
    variations of, 148–149, 195
pressure-free eating, 25, 38–39, 52, 71,
    79, 161, 170, 219–220

R

reflux, 49–50, 78
regression, in eating, 19, 77–78, 133, 152–123, 158–159, 190
roles in feeding, 117–118, 152, 219–220, 226–227
routines, meal, 18, 26, 68, 109, 117, 139, 142–144, 160–164, 188–189, 217

S

safety, at mealtime, 17, 114–115, 167, 225–226
Satter, Ellyn, 9, 117, 136, 162, 219
schedule, eating, 69–70, 134–138, 140–141, 162, 222–223, 226
school, eating at, 22–23, 98, 105–108, 110–113, 128, 174
screens, at meals, 25–26, 81–86, 113, 193–194, 221
self-feeding, 17, 24, 81, 85, 189–190
sensory exploration, 17, 28–29, 60–61, 145, 238
sensory processing impairments, 19, 51–52, 58–59, 92, 159, 185–187
Sequential Oral Sensory (SOS) Approach to Feeding. See sensory exploration
serving meals, 73, 120–121, 149, 224–225
serving sizes, 225
shared meals. See family meals, shared
shopping. See grocery shopping
siblings, 143, 175
sight, of food, as displeasing, 185
smell, 30–32, 52, 59, 122, 130–131, 185–186, 199, 211, 227
snacks
    frequency of, 69–70, 134–135, 222
    introducing new food at, 231
    planning, 144–145
    processed/packaged, 16, 20, 133
    scheduled, 140–141, 222–223
social implications, 16, 25, 27–28, 40, 105–106, 166–167, 192
sound, of food, 30–31, 59, 227–228
special needs children, 8, 53, 77, 83–84, 92, 158, 185–186. See also sensory processing impairments
spectrum disorders. See autism/spectrum disorders
structure, meals. See routines, meal
supertaster, 62–64

T

table, dinner
    comfort and, 142–143, 193
    leaving during meal, 157, 164–165
tactile interaction, 130–131, 211, 228
taste
    changes in and dietary deficiencies, 191
    describing, 32, 65, 146
    development of, 23–24, 97–98
    dips masking, 176–177
    flavor identification (See under flavors: identification of)
    food introduction and, 123–124
    intensiveness of (See under flavors: intensity)
    quick on tongue/snake test, 32, 42, 198, 212
    science of, 126
    senses, using to explore, 17, 31
    sensitivities, 58
    sensory exploration activities, 36–37, 131–132
    supertaster, 62–64
    Taste Test, 36–37, 39, 47–48
teenagers, 22
textures, 23, 33, 168, 176
tolerance, 29, 66, 188–189, 238
Toomey, Kay, 9, 24, 29, 90, 95, 122, 144, 200
touch, as sense exploration, 130–131, 211, 228
tracking foods, 234, 245

U

utensil usage, 80–81, 152, 189

V

vitamin deficiencies/multivitamins, 83–84, 191–192

W

weight concerns, 49–51, 69–71, 82, 143, 187–188, 226, 229